Behavioral Approaches
to Cardiovascular Disease

BEHAVIORAL MEDICINE

Series Editors:

Richard S. Surwit
Redford B. Williams, Jr.
Department of Psychiatry
Duke University Medical Center
Durham, North Carolina

David Shapiro
Department of Psychiatry
University of California, Los Angeles
Los Angeles, California

Robert Ader (Ed.): *Psychoneuroimmunology*

Joel F. Lubar and William M. Deering: *Behavioral Approaches to Neurology*

Richard S. Surwit, Redford B. Williams, Jr., and David Shapiro: *Behavioral Approaches to Cardiovascular Disease*

Behavioral Approaches to Cardiovascular Disease

RICHARD S. SURWIT

REDFORD B. WILLIAMS, JR.
Behavioral Physiology Laboratory
Department of Psychiatry
Duke University Medical Center
Durham, North Carolina

DAVID SHAPIRO
Department of Psychiatry
School of Medicine
University of California, Los Angeles
Los Angeles, California

ACADEMIC PRESS   1982
A Subsidiary of Harcourt Brace Jovanovich, Publishers
New York   London
Paris   San Diego   San Francisco   São Paulo
Sydney   Tokyo   Toronto

The writing of this book was supported in part by
National Institute of Mental Health, Research Scientists
Development Awards, No. MH 00303 to Richard S. Surwit
and MH 18589 to Redford B. Williams, Jr.

ACADEMIC PRESS, INC.
111 Fifth Avenue, New York, New York 10003

United Kingdom Edition published by
ACADEMIC PRESS, INC. (LONDON) LTD.
24/28 Oval Road, London NW1   7DX

Library of Congress Cataloging in Publication Data

Surwit, Richard S.
    Behavioral approaches to cardiovascular disease.

    (Behavioral medicine series)
    Includes bibliographies and index.
    1. Cardiovascular system--Diseases--Psychological
aspects. 2. Behavior therapy. 3. Medicine and
psychology. I. Williams, Redford Brown, Date.
II. Shapiro, David, Date. III. Title. IV. Series.
[DNLM: 1. Cardiovascular diseases. 2. Behavior
therapy. 3. Cardiovascular system--physiopathology.
WG 166 S963b]
RC669.S86   616.1'0651   81-17635
ISBN 0-12-677480-3   AACR2

PRINTED IN THE UNITED STATES OF AMERICA

82 83 84 85   9 8 7 6 5 4 3 2 1

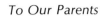

To Our Parents

Contents

1

Introduction   1

2

Measurement of Cardiovascular Function:
A Brief Overview   9

3

Introduction to Cardiovascular Psychophysiology   23

4

Conditioning and Learning of Cardiovascular Functions   61

5

Coronary Heart Disease   87

6

Hypertension   129

7

Raynaud's Disease and Raynaud's Phenomenon   157

.

Introduction to the Series

Behavioral Medicine is an emerging field which has undergone nearly explosive growth in the past 5 years. In 1977, the National Institutes of Health sponsored a conference on Behavioral Medicine at Yale University. The conference adopted the following definition of behavioral medicine: "Behavioral Medicine is an interdisciplinary field concerned with the integration of behavioral and biomedical science knowledge and techniques relevant to health and disease and the application of this knowledge and these techniques to prevention treatment and rehabilitation."

The books in this series will provide a medium for the presentation, in depth, of research findings on various topics falling within the domain of Behavioral Medicine. Each will contain careful reviews of the scientific evidence relevant to each of the specific topic areas. Most volumes will be written by a team of behavioral and biomedical scientists.

This series will constitute a growing and evolving archive documenting the scientific basis of Behavioral Medicine. As such, its intended audience is broad—ranging from basic research scientists to practicing clinicians.

R.S.S.
R.B.W.
D.S.
Series Editors

Preface

Behavioral Medicine is broadly defined to encompass the application of principles from all behavioral sciences to medical problems. Behavioral Medicine has applied behavioral science to the understanding of etiology and pathogenesis as well as to the development of behavioral procedures useful in the treatment and rehabilitation of disease. In perhaps no other area is the evidence of the applicability of behavioral science to disease so extensive and convincing as it is in cardiovascular disease. *Behavioral Approaches to Cardiovascular Disease* was conceived as a timely review of this important and growing field.

Coronary heart disease and hypertension and its complications account for more than three times the deaths attributable to all forms of cancer in the United States each year. Recent findings have led to the conclusion that Type A (coronary-prone) behavior pattern is a major risk factor for heart disease—one of about the same magnitude as such well known risk factors as high blood pressure, serum cholesterol, and cigarette smoking. In the following chapters, we will review in detail the contributions of behavioral science to the understanding of coronary heart disease. Separate chapters will examine the measurement of cardiovascular function, basic principles of cardiovascular psychophysiology, conditioning and learning of cardiovascular functions, and the behavioral variables relevant to the pathogenesis and treatment of coronary heart disease.

Although the role of behavioral factors in the pathogenesis of other cardiovascular disorders is not as clear, it is now apparent that behavioral techniques have a role to play in the management of many forms of cardiovascular disease. The new field of Behavioral Medicine has applied the technology of behavior modification to the treatment of many disorders whose pathogenesis is thought to be purely physical. Research over the last 20 years has demonstrated that learning techniques can be used to teach patients voluntary control of a variety of autonomically mediated functions. These self-control procedures are now being widely applied to the treatment of hypertension, peripheral vascular disease, and chronic headaches. Furthermore, behavioral procedures are now being used to improve adherence to medical treatment regimens. This is extremely important in the treatment of hypertension, in which the failure of patients to adhere to prescribed antihypertensive medical regiments has been identified as the major problem in treatment. The latter part of this book deals with the specific applications of behavioral procedures in the treatment of hypertension, peripheral vascular disease, and vascular headache. The concluding chapter reviews the important clinical considerations involved in the application of behavioral principles to the treatment of disease, including a discussion on enhancing adherence to conventional treatment regimens.

Behavioral Approaches to Cardiovascular Disease presents, in a concise monograph form, a complete review of the state of knowledge of cardiovascular behavioral medicine. Both the clinical and experimental literature are critically surveyed. Thus, the book should be of major interest to both scientists and practitioners interested in learning about the contributions of behavioral science to cardiovascular disease, and of significant interest to medical and graduate students as well.

ACKNOWLEDGMENTS

We wish to express our appreciation to our colleagues and students who contributed in many different ways to this book. In several chapters we adopted material from previously published reviews written in collaboration with our associates. Special thanks are extended to James A. Blumenthal, Iris B. Goldstein, W. Doyle Gentry, J. Alberto Mainardi, and John L. Reeves.

1

Introduction

Behavioral Medicine refers to a major new development in the behavioral sciences and medicine that involves a radical change from the usual approach of medicine today. It is part of a movement which will significantly alter the course of health research and the everyday practice of medicine. Like many new successful ideas, the rapid development of behavioral medicine is due to the simultaneous occurrence of a demand for innovation and the presence of a new technology that seems suited to the demand.

There is an increasing realization of the inadequacies of the present health-care system. The cost of the health care is growing without an accompanying improvement in health.[1] In 1950, Americans spent 4.6% of the Gross National Product for health care. Twenty-five years later, in 1975, the percentage increased to 8.3%. Medical care is one of the largest industries in the United States. But further expansion of present medicine does not seem warranted. It has been estimated that a doubling of medical expenditures for the current system of medical care would have little impact on longevity. There is also a growing awareness of and concern about the negative consequences of certain current medical practices, such as the injurious effects of the misuse and overuse of drugs and medications and the complications of unnecessary or undesirable surgery. It is disturbing to realize how little we know about the possible adverse consequences of long-term use of many drugs. The message at present seems to be *restraint* in the current practice of medicine—to do less, to justify what is done, and to attempt to reorient and restructure our system of medical care in a more positive direction. In 1974, the Canadian government published a document called "A New Perspective on the Health of Canadians." It was prompted by the fact that universal free medical care in Canada has had no real impact on mortality rates. The report concludes that methods for deal-

[1]See O. F. Pomerleau and J. P. Brady (Eds.) *Behavioral medicine: theory and practice.* Baltimore: Williams and Wilkins Co., 1979.

ing with lifestyle and environmental influences on health be given the same prominence in the field of health as hospitals, clinics, and private physicians. Similarly, in 1979, the United States Department of Health, Education and Welfare issued a report entitled, "*Promoting Health, Preventing Disease: Objectives for the Nation,*" which concluded that behavior and environmental influences may be related to the pathophysiology of numerous diseases and that a comprehensive treatment approach should include multiple behavioral inputs. Behavioral Medicine stresses behavioral factors not only as they relate to the etiology and pathogenesis of disease but also to the prevention of disease, the maintenance and promotion of good health, and an increased utilization of behavioral approaches in treatment.

BEHAVIORAL VERSUS PSYCHOSOMATIC MEDICINE

To understand what is new about "behavioral medicine," it is necessary to consider how it differs from the field that has traditionally concerned itself with the relationship between emotion and illness—psychosomatic medicine. Psychosomatic medicine began with the study of psychological factors in seven disorders that were considered to be psychosomatic: duodenal ulcer, asthma, Graves's disease, essential hypertension, ulcerative colitis, neurodermatitis, and rheumatoid arthritis. The primary focus was on specific personality traits which it was felt, led to neurotic conflicts that were in some way responsible for the emergence of the disease in question. This focus on intrapsychic conflicts determined that therapeutic interventions focused on the spontaneous verbal productions of the patient, with the goal of achieving insights that would hopefully result in the amelioration of the disease process.

The major differences between the behavioral model and the psychosomatic model are depicted in Figure 1.1. A patient presents with a disease or a set of isolated physical symptoms. According to the psychosomatic model, this physiologic disturbance is directly traceable to a neurotic conflict. The neurotic conflict in turn seems to be rooted in the disorder of the personality. Notice that both the neurotic conflict and the personality disorder are hypothetical constructs, the presence of which are based on inferred data. In contrast, the behavioral model dissects the patient's problem into changes in behavior and/or physiology. These changes can be determined from observable data that can be quantified. Whereas intervention in the psychosomatic approach is directed at a hypothetical problem, behavioral intervention is aimed at changing behavior and/or physiology directly. The effectiveness of this change is readily assessable through behavioral observation and conventional techniques of physiological monitoring.

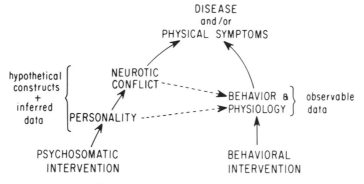

FIGURE 1.1. Psychosomatic and behavioral models of disease intervention.

The emerging technology of Behavioral Medicine comes from research on biofeedback and behavior therapy. The first significant use of the term *Behavioral Medicine* occurred in a book on biofeedback published in 1973, edited by Lee Birk. It contained articles describing clinical applications of biofeedback techniques to various disorders. The book was entitled *Biofeedback: Behavioral Medicine,* a title that called attention to the fact that biofeedback and related behavioral techniques may be viewed as behavior therapy or behavior modification for the control of physical symptoms of medical disorders.

Biofeedback or operant conditioning is one of two major methods, the other being classical or Pavlovian conditioning, for the study of learned or acquired change in physiology and behavior as a function of experience, particularly as related to temporal associations of stimuli in the environment. These conditioning methods constitute the most systematic and productive means that have been devised by behavioral scientists for generating information about the plasticity of behavioral and physiological adjustment to stimuli or situations. The methods provide a means of describing, predicting, and controlling transient or permanent modifications of behavior occurring as a consequence of experience—*the phenomena of learning.* These procedures, which are reviewed in detail in Chapter 4, are used to control or regulate covert physiological responses in the same way that other behavioral procedures are applied to overt behaviors. They are also used to control physical symptoms of disease in more or less the same fashion as other methods of conditioning or learning are used to manage symptoms of behavioral disorders.

The following are the main characteristics of a behavioral approach to treatment:

1. The behavioral approach does not rely upon psychodynamic labels to diagnose or treat patients. Rather, the behavior or physiological response

in question is studied empirically and described as a function of its relationship to environmental events. Instead of questioning whether or not a specific problem is psychosomatic, psychogenic, or physiological, the behavioral approach determines whether the presenting symptoms may be treated by manipulating behavior and/or environment.

2. The behavioral approach relies largely on the experimental principles of learning as the basis of treatment. Though the principles of classical conditioning and operant conditioning are emphasized, the modern behavioral approach draws heavily upon principles from experimental and social psychology. The importance of cognitive events and symbolic learning are recognized and utilized.

3. The behavioral approach involves the specification of replicable treatment procedures and the objective evaluation of therapeutic outcome. Both behavioral and physiological data are collected during baseline treatment and follow-up periods.

Several factors are responsible for the striking emergence of Behavioral Medicine as a distinct field of endeavor in recent years. First is the realization that, except for those few patients with clear evidence of clinically significant neurotic conflicts, most patients with physical disease have not been shown to benefit with regard to their specific physical disease problem from the application of psychodynamically oriented therapy that focused upon verbal productions and free associations with the goal of achieving insight. Second, and probably more important, has been (a) the discovery in large-scale epidemiological studies that certain behaviors or lifestyles are "risk factors" for usch major physical disorders as cancer and coronary heart disease; and (b) the realization on the part of some leaders in clinical medicine that behavior modification approaches, effective in changing behavior associated with mental disorders, might also prove useful in attempts to modify behaviors that are risk factors for major physical disorders. Third is the demonstration in a growing body of clinical research that behavioral treatment approaches are effective in the treatment of such physical disorders as headache, chronic pain, and Raynaud's disease—disorders that heretofore had proven unusually resistant to the application of the traditional approaches of biomedicine.

What is attractive about the broad concept of *Behavioral Medicine* then is first the availability of specific techniques derived from behavioral research for the direct control or alleviation of physical symptoms of disease. Second is the reliance on objective definitions and measures of behavior and the use of empirically based principles of behavior. Third is its applicability, at least in principle, to *all* medical disorders, rather than only to disorders traditionally defined as purely psychological or psychophysiological in nature. This last point is important from a number of standpoints. Behavioral Medicine, opposes the simplistic organic–functional dichotomy that has tended to define a disease as psychosomatic by excluding physical causes. Essential hypertension is a case in point here, a disease of so-called unknown cause. Yet, clearly, we know that alterations of the functions of the heart, blood vessels, and kidneys are subject to behavioral regulation and to neurogenic dysfunction. The causes are there for us to see if we look and study them. Behavioral processes can in principle enter into any disease process, although they may function in different ways in different phases of each disease. Behavioral Medicine keeps open the possibility of behavioral processes contributing to what are assumed to be purely physical diseases, either to their pathogenesis or to their treatment, and, similarly, of biological processes contributing to what are assumed to be purely psychological disorders.

It is interesting that the behavioral approach to disease probably comes closer than any other psychological method to the approach of conventional medicine in which a treatment can be rationally devised to deal directly with a symptom. One behavioral technique, biofeedback, may be viewed as akin to the use of specific drugs to correct a deficiency or control a symptom. This involves tapping into neural processes of regulation by behavioral means. This feature derives from basic research in biofeedback that shows that specific responses or patterns of response can be modified by biofeedback techniques. In biofeedback research on the cardiovascular system, for example, it has been shown that selective control can be achieved over particular cardiovascular responses or patterns of response. Thus, clinically, one can select appropriate indices for feedback and self-regulation. In labile hypertension, characterized by increased cardiac output, feedback training to achieve a decreased heart rate or for a combined pattern of heart rate and blood pressure decrease, decreased muscle blood flow, and increased skin blood flow might be selected. In the case of fixed hypertension, in which total peripheral resistance is elevated, feedback for decreases in diastolic pressure would be in order. It may be useful to look carefully at drug treatment in hypertension and examine parallels between specific drug interventions and possible parallels in a behavioral intervention. The Stepped Care Approach (Report of the Joint National Committee on detection, evaluation, and treatment of high blood pressure, 1977) is used in drug therapy for hypertension. Treatment usually starts with a diuretic. Sympathetic nervous system blocking agents, and certain vasodilator agents are added sequentially, if necessary. What would be parallels in behavioral procedures? Decrease heart rate biofeedback training would be a possible substitute for propranolol, a beta blocking agent. Vasodilation training using blood flow or blood volume feedback would be a parallel to the use of vasodilator drugs. In an example of another cardiovascular disease in the management of patients with ischemic heart disease whose anginal attacks are often related to emotional events, the learned ability to minimize an episode of tachycardia might be helpful, in an analogous maneuver to propranolol.

INDIVIDUAL DIFFERENCES, LIFE-STYLE, AND SOCIAL CULTURAL FACTORS

As suggested earlier, however, *disease* needs to be thought of in the context of behavioral, social, and environmental factors. Behavioral Medicine, although it was stimulated by the developments in biofeedback, relaxation, and related technique, concerns the whole spectrum of behavioral and environmental factors involved in health and disease. These include behavioral processes and habits that may enter directly into the chain of causation or remediation or disease, such as smoking, overeating, alcohol intake, specific dietary factors (e.g., sodium and cholesterol), and exercise and physical activity. Such behaviors are not the immediate causes of diseases, but they are just as clearly risk factors as are the specific physical abnormalities. Of further concern are behaviors involving response to threat and stress, or adaptation to change and disruption in daily life adjustments. We talk about these factors in such terms as anxiety, feelings of helplessness or frustration, depression, and difficulties of coping and adaptation. The concept of *stress* has been used to refer to the stimuli or events that are the presumed source of maladaptive behavioral and physiological reactions as well as to the specific and nonspecific effects of such stimuli on the individual. One can point to pain, punishment, demanding mental effort, sustained work, or behaviors requiring continuous adjustments. Even relatively commonplace behaviors such as exercise, postural change, feeding, and sexual activity can have a potent influence on cardiovascular and other functions. However, noxious environmental events may not by themselves determine adverse reactions. Rather, the outcome often depends upon how the person perceives the source of the stress, and how the person sees his own capacity to cope with the stress. Richard Lazarus (1977) advanced the concept of *cognitive appraisal* to characterize the psychological context of the emotion arising from adaptive transactions between the individual and the environment. Cognitive appraisal "expresses the evaluation of the significance of a transaction for the person's well-being and the potentials for mastery in the continuous and constantly changing interplay between the person and the environmental stimulus configuration [p. 15]."

Another method of related study involves individual differences; the best current example being identification of the Type A coronary-prone behavior pattern characterized by such behavioral attributes as impatience, time urgency, competitiveness, excessive activity, and aggressiveness (Rosenman, Friedman, and Strauss, 1964). The Type A behavioral pattern is clearly associated with coronary heart disease, atherosclerosis, and recurrent heart attacks.

This research on Type A behavior stands in sharp contrast to psychosomatic research aimed at identifying underlying personality patterns and neurotic processes responsible for disease. The primary focus of attention in the Type A research was on overt manifest behavior exhibited by the subjects; a focus which led to the employment of a structured interview with close observation of speech stylistics and psychomotor mannerisms. No doubt the investigators studying Type A behavior pattern in relation to coronary artery disease at times drew inferences concerning possible underlying personality characteristics. However, this was never the primary focus.

Indeed, the emergence of Behavioral Medicine as a distinct field was heralded at the Timberline Conference on Psychophysiologic Aspects of Cardiovascular Disease in 1964 when Rosenman made the following response to those who criticized the Type A behavior pattern concept as inadequate because it did not attempt to define "important traits in a personality" which could be related to disease processes:

> We have not concerned ourselves with factors of motivation but only with determining the presence or absence of the *overt* pattern A, and I suspect that (those objecting to absence of concern with personality traits) are upset at this as well as our seeming oversimplification of inexact factors that are difficult to assess and even more difficult to quantitate.... (however) it is possible... to study different aspects of men that are tall and men that are short... without determining why they are tall or short [p. 429].

Documentation of the utility of this focus on overt behavior in the emerging field of Behavioral Medicine is provided by the conclusion of a blue ribbon panel of behavioral and biomedical scientists recently convened by the NHLBI that the Type A behavior pattern is associated with increased risk of developing coronary heart disease. This increased risk is over and above that imposed by age, systolic blood pressure, serum cholesterol, and smoking, and appears to be of the same order of magnitude as the relative risk of these physical factors. The realization that no specific intrapsychic conflict has ever been so assessed as a risk factor for any major disease entity is one reason why Behavioral Medicine has incited much more interest among medical researchers than the old psychosomatic model.

Thus, Behavioral Medicine has assimilated time-honored concerns about the role of individual differences, life-style, and social–cultural factors with more recent developments in specific methods of self-regulation and self-control involving biofeedback and conditioning, relaxation, various forms of self-monitoring and self-management, along with the total armamentarium of behavior modification.

REFERENCES

A new perspective on the health of Canadians: A working paper (Marc LaLonde). Ottawa Government of Canada, 1974.

Birk, L. (Ed.). *Biofeedback: Behavioral medicine,* New York: Grune and Statton, 1973.

Lazarus, R. S. Psychological stress and coping in adaptation and illness. In. Z. J. Lipowski, D. R. Lipsitt, & P. C. Whybrow (Eds.), *Psychosomatic medicine: Current trends and clinical applications.* New York: Oxford University Press, 1977.

Promoting health, preventing disease: Objectives for the nation. United States Department of Health, Education and Welfare, 1979.

Rosenman, R. H., Friedman, M., Strauss, R., *et al* A predictive study of coronary heart disease: The Western Collaborative Group Study. *Journal of the American Medical Association,* 1964, *189,* 15–22.

The Stepped Care Approach. Report of the Joint National Committee on detection, evaluation, and treatment of high blood pressure. *Journal of the American Medical Association,* 1977, 237, 255–261.

Timberline conference on psychophysiologic aspects of cardiovascular disease. *Psychosomatic Medicine,* 1964, 26, 405–541.

2

Measurement of Cardiovascular Function: A Brief Overview

The first and essential step to be taken by anyone contemplating any study of cardiovascular function is to gain some understanding of the basic physiology of the cardiovascular system. Both the novice just starting out and the old hand wishing to refresh his or her understanding of basic principles would be well advised to undertake a close perusal of the excellent text by Folkow and Neil (1971). Although an exhaustive review of this topic would be beyond the scope of this brief overview, we shall review certain basic principles of cardiovascular organization that are essential for any rational approach to issues of measurement of cardiovascular function. With these principles in mind, we shall next move to a consideration of a selected number of techniques for quantification of various aspects of cardiovascular system functioning—particularly those of use to the psychophysiologist. Finally, we shall conclude with a brief overview of some of the analytic issues involved in interpreting data obtained through the use of these techniques.

BASIC PRINCIPLES OF CARDIOVASCULAR PHYSIOLOGY

The first, and simplest, principle to consider is that the function of the cardiovascular system is directed toward one central purpose: meeting the metabolic needs of the various tissues that make up the body. This involves both the delivery of oxygen, nutrients, and other vital substances (e.g., electrolytes and vitamins) to tissues and the removal of wastes. It follows, therefore, that the key aspect of the total cardiovascular system's functioning, to which all other aspects are subservient, is maintenance of a rate of *flow* of blood to tissues

9

consistent with their particular needs. Although this first principle is simple, the means by which the cardiovascular system functions in an integrated fashion to meet the metabolic needs of the various body tissues is exceedingly complex. This complexity is illustrated in Figure 2.1, which shows the variations in cardiac output and distribution of that output under conditions of rest and heavy physical exercise.

The cardiac output is the product of the heart rate and the stroke volume of each heartbeat and varies over a wide range, from about 5 liters per minute at rest to 25 liters per minute during heavy exercise. As shown in Figure 2.1, the distribution of this output to the vascular beds serving various organs also shows marked variations. For example, during rest about 50% of the total cardiac output is going to the renal and mesenteric circuits and only 15% is going to skeletal muscles. In contrast, during heavy work only about 8–10% of the blood pumped by the heart is distributed to the mesenteric and renal vascular beds, while a full 80% goes to the exercising skeletal muscle. As we

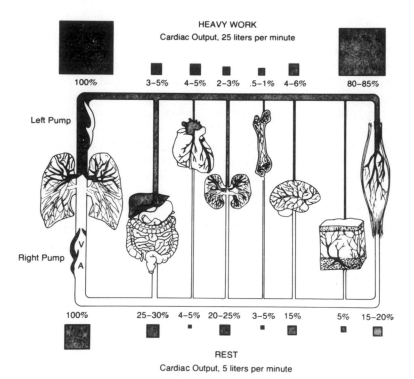

FIGURE 2.1. Distribution of cardiac output during heavy work and rest. [From J. Hassett, *A primer of psychophysiology*. (San Francisco: Freeman, 1978, p. 52).]

shall see in Chapter 3, which deals with cardiovascular psychophysiology, similar shifts occur in association with varying behavioral states.

These changes in cardiac output and its varying distribution to various bodily tissues occur through the action of a broad array of mechanisms ranging in locus from the cerebral cortex to the cellular level in the tissues themselves. To a large extent, the hypothalamus and brain stem function as an integrating center for neurogenic cardiovascular control mechanisms, the efferent limb of which involves changes in sympathetic and parasympathetic outflow. To make the picture even more complex, there is also provision for extensive afferent feedback to the brain of information about what is happening in the cardiovascular system. This afferent feedback has its origin in mechanoreceptors, pressoreceptors, and chemoreceptors scattered throughout the body. This afferent feedback serves to modulate the efferent outflow.

While any detailed consideration of these various control mechanisms would be clearly beyond the scope of this chapter, a consideration of some of the mechanisms controlling two important aspects of cardiovascular function— cardiac output and blood flow to skeletal muscle—will serve as illustration.

As just noted, the cardiac output is the product of the rate at which the heart is beating and the volume of blood ejected with each heartbeat. The heart rate, in turn, is determined by the balance between the parasympathetic (cholinergic) and sympathetic (adrenergic) innervations of the heart. Stimulation of the vagal parasympathetic input results in slowing of the heart rate, and stimulation of the cardiac sympathetic nerves results in speeding. With regard to net control of heart rate, however, the parasympathetic innervation appears to be capable of overriding the sympathetic input, such that stimulation of both inputs would still result in slowing. In addition, as heart rate increases, the rate of firing of the baroreceptor cells in the carotid sinus increases, with subsequent increased afferent input to the nucleus tractus solitarius in the brain stem, resulting in increased vagal outflow to slow the heart rate. The operation of this baroreceptor reflex is not a simple stimulus–response linkage, however. When the heart rate (and cardiac output) increases as a result of activation of the hypothalamic defense reaction (see Chapter 3), the baroreceptor reflex is damped, such that increased vagal output does not occur and the heart rate remains elevated.

The factors determining the stroke volume of blood ejected with each heartbeat are similarly complex. Basically, stroke volume depends on the *preload* and *afterload*. Preload depends on the rate of return of blood via the venous system to the heart. If the total blood volume in the body is decreased, the rate of venous return will be low. If the venous system is dilated, blood will be pooled in this reservoir, and venous return and, hence, cardiac output will be diminished; on the other hand, with venoconstriction the venous return and cardiac output will increase. Afterload is essentially the resistance in the arterial system that the heart must overcome in order to pump blood. This is determined by the net resistance resulting from the parallel resistances of all the various vascular beds. In addition to their direct influences on the amount of blood available for the heart to eject with each beat and the resistance to each ejection, preload and afterload also act to influence stroke volume indirectly, via mechanisms intrinsic to cardiac muscle function. Because of an increased stretching of cardiac muscle fibers with increased preload, the force of contraction of the muscle increases (Starling's "Law of the Heart") and stroke volume rises concomitantly. Increased afterload, with its attendant increase in aortic blood pressure, also results in increased myocardial contractility via the mechanism of *homeometric ventricular autoregulation* (Sarnoff, Mitchell, Gilmore, & Remensnyder, 1960).

Let us turn now to a consideration of the determinants of blood flow in the skeletal muscle vascular bed. Independently of the cardiac output, skeletal muscle blood flow can increase and decrease via mechanisms that are both active and passive. Muscle blood flow decreases actively via increased sympathetic nerve stimulation of alpha receptors in arterial smooth muscle, and beta-adrenergic stimulation by circulating epinephrine results in an active vasodilatation in the muscle vascular bed. Withdrawal of either of these sources of active vasoconstriction or vasodilatation results in passive vasodilatation or vasoconstriction, respectively. Thus, there are at least two neurogenic or hormonal mechanisms whereby either increased or decreased muscle blood flow can be brought about. In addition, with increased muscle work the production of lactic acid as a metabolic product results in a vasodilatation via local effects that act to overcome any neurogenic vasoconstrictor effects. Finally, when the blood flow to muscle is in excess of its metabolic needs, as might occur during mental work via increased circulating epinephrine (see Chapter 3), local autoregulatory mechanisms come into play to decrease the rate of blood flow to be more consistent with metabolic needs.

This illustrative overview of selected cardiovascular control mechanisms by no means exhausts what is known of cardiovascular regulation, and there is much more that is still not known. It should be clear, however, that anyone wishing to study cardiovascular–behavioral relationships would be sorely misguided in attempting to define the influence of any specific behavior on a single aspect of cardiovascular function in the absence of any consideration of the complex interrelationships among all aspects of cardiovascular function, which are only touched upon here. For example, blood pressure is a variable that has long attracted the interest of psychophysiological investigators. By now the reader should realize, however, that blood pressure does not even exist as a primary function. It is determined by the product of the cardiac output and total peripheral resistance, and these, in turn, are complexly determined, as illustrated in the preceeding discussion. As we shall see in Chapter 3, there are qualitatively different mechanisms whereby behavioral influences can act to increase blood pressure. On the one hand, there is increased blood pressure due primarily to increased cardiac output; on the other, there is increased blood pressure due primarily to increased total peripheral resistance. If one is only measuring blood pressure, it is obvious that one will be unable to determine which of these two possible mechanisms is responsible for the increase in blood pressure observed in response to some behavioral challenge. Similarly, if one is studying that favorite variable of the psychophysiologist, heart rate, in isolation of a consideration of what is happening in the rest of the cardiovascular system, one will have at best an incomplete understanding of what is actually happening. At worst, one will be seriously misled. With the foregoing in mind, we shall now turn to a consideration of what one would want to measure and how one would do it in any rational approach to a study of cardiovascular psychophysiology.

TECHNIQUES OF CARDIOVASCULAR MEASUREMENT

While blood pressure and heart rate are relatively easy to measure using noninvasive techniques, it is important to remember that it is maintenance of blood flow that is the primary function of the cardiovascular system. When one is measuring heart rate and blood pressure, one should keep in mind that one is merely sampling indirect measures of the cardiovascular system's attempt to maintain appropriate blood flow to body tissues.

In this section, we shall review only noninvasive techniques for the study of cardiovascular function, since these are the ones most often available to those interested in studying behavioral–cardiovascular relationships. We shall not go into the basics of electrophysiological recording, for which the reader is referred to the texts by Hassett (1978) and Stern, Ray, and Davis (1980). Other basic manuals of psychophysiological and bioelectric recording techniques supply detailed information on fundamentals of physiological instrumentation and electronic circuitry that are particularly relevant to behavioral research, along with a consideration of issues of response quantification and analysis (Brown, 1967; Martin & Venables, 1980; Thompson, & Patterson, 1974; Venables & Martin, 1967).

Whole body blood flow is the same as the cardiac output. Within the range of normal heart rates, from 50–60 to 140–150 beats per min, heart rate and cardiac output are reasonably well correlated. Thus, an indirect measure of cardiac output can be obtained by simply measuring the heart rate from the electrocardiogram (EKG). To obtain an *absolute* measure of cardiac output, one must resort to invasive measures, such as dye-dilution. The noninvasive technique of impedance cardiography is based on the principle that the impedance to passage of an alternating electric current passed across electrodes placed on the chest in an appropriate configuration varies as a function of the amount of blood pumped with each heartbeat. This technique provides a *relative* measure of cardiac output; that is, with the same subject within a single experimental session, it is possible to measure accurately relative changes in cardiac output from one experimental condition or baseline period to the next. These changes can be expressed only as relative or proportional changes, however, and comparisons across individuals with regard to absolute levels of cardiac output are not possible with impedance cardiography.

If we consider measurement of blood flow in the various vascular beds, rather than whole body blood flow, a number of noninvasive techniques are available. Most of these again provide information with regard only to relative changes; however, one method, venous occlusion plethysmography, does permit noninvasisve measurement of absolute rates of blood flow in certain bodily parts and will be described in some detail.

A number of techniques permit the measurement of relative changes in skin blood flow. Perhaps, the most widely used technique is photoelectric plethysmography. Because the light reflectance of skin varies mainly as a function of changes in blood volume with each heartbeat, a photocell can be employed to measure this reflected light (provided by a separate light source) and, hence, provide a measure of skin blood flow. Since the temperature on the skin surface varies as a function of blood flow through the skin, simple monitoring of the skin temperature using a thermistor also provides an indirect measure of skin blood flow. For a more detailed overview of the issues involved in the measurement of skin blood flow, the reader is referred to papers by Cook (1974) and Jennings, Tahmaush, and Redmond (1980).

As noted earlier, the skeletal muscle vascular bed shows the greatest variation in the range of blood flow that it receives as a percentage of the cardiac output under various conditions. The technique of venous occlusion plethysmography is an established method that has been used for several decades to provide an absolute measure of blood flow in the arm or leg. Forearm blood flow (FBF) is made up of blood flow to muscle, skin, and bone. Under resting conditions the proportion of the FBF distributed to muscle is in the range of 70–80%, whereas with exercise this proportion becomes even greater. Thus, measurement of FBF is generally considered to provide a fairly accurate index of skeletal muscle blood flow.

Although water-filled volumetric plethysmographs have been used to measure FBF in association with venous occlusion, these devices not only are cumbersome and prone to a wide variety of leakage problems but also require long-term immobilization of the arm, even when measurements are not being taken. Whitney (1953) documented the validity of strain gauge plethysmography as a means of detecting changes in limb volume in association with venous occlusion, and most laboratories now measuring FBF on a regular basis use this technique. The necessary components of a system to measure FBF are illustrated in Figure 2.2. A mercury-in-silastic (or rubber) strain gauge (component 10 in Figure 2.2) is placed around the largest circumference of the forearm (where the ratio of muscle to skin and bone is greatest) and attached to a suitable Wheatstone Bridge-type circuit (e.g., Parks Model 270® Plethysmograph) (11 in Figure 2.2) to provide a means of recording small changes in the electrical resistance of the mercury column. As illustrated by Whitney (1953), it is possible to use a device for mounting the strain gauge on the arm that also contains a movable element. By turning a screw, it is possible to actually stretch the strain gauge a known fixed amount (e.g., 1mm), thus calibrating the gauge with respect to its balanced state for the sensitivity setting of the amplifier feeding into the recorder. This setup provides a plethsymographic tracing that varies directly with the volume of the limb. With a (DC) recording technique, the pulsations with each beat are readily seen, as well as more long-lived changes in arm circumference, as with venous occlusion.

To determine FBF, it is also necessary to have two blood pressure cuffs, one placed around the wrist (8 in Figure 2.2) and one around the upper arm (9 in Figure 2.2), proximal to the strain gauge (10 in Figure 2.2). Prior to venous occlusion, the wrist cuff is inflated to a pressure greater than systolic (e.g., 200 mm Hg). It is necessary to thus exclude the hand circulation from

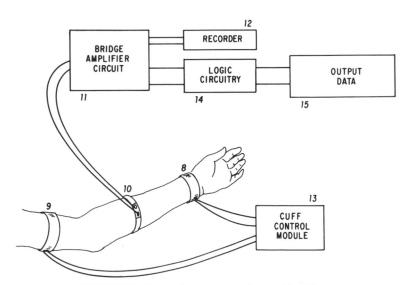

FIGURE 2.2. System for measuring forearm blood flow.

the measurement field because, in contrast to the forearm, the blood flow to the hand is largely determined by skin blood flow. Thus, with the hand circulation included, it is much more difficult to be sure that any changes in flow measured in the forearm are due to muscle rather than skin blood flow. Before this was known, a number of studies were carried out with widely varying results. This is because, in contrast to muscle with its active mechanisms for both vasoconstriction and vasodilatation, the skin has neurogenic mechanisms only subserving vasoconstriction. Neurogenic vasodilatation in skin occurs only passively, as a result of sympathetic withdrawal.

Once the hand circulation is excluded, the next step in FBF measurement is simply to inflate the upper arm cuff quickly to a pressure that is above venous pressure but below diastolic arterial pressure. In practice, an occlusion pressure of about 50 mm Hg is generally used. This maneuver does not affect the arterial inflow to the arm, but it does block the venous outflow. Consequently, the arm begins to enlarge, and a *venous occlusion slope* is generated on the plethysmographic recording (12 in Figure 2.2), the rate of rise of which is directly proportional to the rate of increase in arm circumference. Since the volume increase of the forearm with venous occlusion occurs in terms only of circumference and not in the length of the arm, the rate of increase in limb circumference with venous occlusion is a direct measure of the rate of arterial inflow—the FBF. To compute FBF from the venous occlusion slope, one draws a line along the linear portion of the slope and extrapolates to determine the rate of rise (usually in millimeters) in the tracing that would occur in 1 min. This number is then divided by the rise in the tracing caused by the calibration procedure (usually stretching the gauge by 1 mm). This gives the actual amount of change in arm circumference that would have occurred in 1 min. By dividing this number by the circumference of the arm at the point of strain gauge placement and multiplying by 100, one obtains the percentage change in arm circumference per minute (%DC/min). Since it can be shown mathematically that the percentage change in *volume* of a cylinder that enlarges by increasing its circumference but not its length can be accurately approximated by twice the percentage change in circumference, one now has only to multiply %DC by two to obtain the percentage change in arm volume per minute (%DV/min). The term %DV/min can also be expressed as cc/100 cc of arm/min—that is, the FBF. Thus, without ever measuring any volume of the arm, it is possible using this approach to determine an index of the rate of change in arm volume corrected for variations across individuals in the volume of their arms. This enables the investigator measuring FBF to state with some confidence that this person who has an FBF of 4 cc/100 cc/min has exactly twice the absolute rate of FBF as someone with an FBF of 2 cc/100 cc/min. In laboratory practice, all these computations can be performed by a small computer (14 and 15 in Figure 2.2).

We have gone into some detail concerning the measurement of FBF because, to our knowledge, it represents virtually the only widely accepted noninvasive measure of absolute flow in an important peripheral vascular bed, that supplying skeletal muscle. When the concomitantly measured mean blood pressure (BP) is divided by the FBF, a direct absolute measure of flow resistance in the forearm is obtained (forearm vascular resistance, FVR = mean BP/FBF). Knowledge of FVR changes enables one to conclude with confidence that vasodilatations or vasoconstrictions observed in the forearm are either active or passive; that is, a significant rise or fall in FVR represents an active vasomotor response. With FBF increasing because of a passive withdrawal of sympathetic vasoconstrictor tone, for example, the blood pressure would also fall, and FVR would be unchanged. As will be documented in Chapter 3, the cardiovascular psychophysiologist armed with this kind of information regarding flow in the cardiovascular system can interpret changes in other parameters (e.g., heart rate and blood pressure) with much more confidence in terms of understanding their place in the patterned response of the cardiovascular system to the various experimental manipulations employed.

Heart rate and blood pressure are the most commonly measured cardiovascular variables in behaviorally oriented studies. Heart rate is assessed simply by counting R-waves in the EKG per unit of time, or changes in rate from beat to beat may be evaluated with a cardiotachometer that reads out proportionately to heart rate. R-waves can be detected automatically with voltage-level devices, and timing devices can be used to obtain a record of each interbeat interval in milliseconds.

Miniaturized and inexpensive electronic devices can be used by any individual to obtain a digital readout in beats per minute of continuous changes in the individual's own heart rate, averaged over two or five beats for example. These are typically finger plethysmographs.

Noninvasive and indirect measurement of blood pressure is a topic of intensive investigation (Tursky, 1974). Along with measures of heart rate and blood flow (described here), blood pressure measurement is also critical to an interpretation of overall cardiovascular functioning. Three broad approaches have been used in the indirect recording of blood pressure in laboratory and clinical studies. The first is an adaptation of the standard method (Riva-Rocci) that can be controlled remotely and automatically. The pressure analog and electronically detected Korotkoff (K) sounds can be recorded on paper. This method can provide a measure of systolic and diastolic pressure roughly once a minute. If either systolic or diastolic levels alone can provide sufficient information, then such a system can be adapted to measure one or the other about three to six times per minute. In measuring systolic, the cuff is inflated to above systolic pressure and gradually deflated until the appearance of the first K-sound. Then the cuff is immediately deflated and, after a brief wait, reinflated and the procedure recycled. In the case of diastolic measurement, the cuff is inflated slowly up to the diastolic pressure level and immediately deflated when the diastolic K-sound is detected. This approach is satisfactory so long as a beat-to-beat continuous measure of pressure is not required. In many research applications, it is desirable to track the continuous progression of cardiovascular change. In biofeedback applications (see Chapters 4 and 6) involving blood pressure, a continuous measure of blood pressure is considered vital, and this necessity led to the development and refinement of other indirect methods.

The first and most widely used method derived from biofeedback research utilizes the constant-cuff principle (Tursky, Shapiro, & Schwartz, 1972). This method involves setting a constant level of pressure in a cuff, above and below which the systolic (or diastolic) blood pressure is expected to vary during the inflation period. The presence, or absence, of a K-sound on a given heartbeat defines an elevation, or reduction, in systolic blood pressure relative to the constant pressure in the cuff. The relation between K-sound and increase or decrease in blood pressure is reversed for diastolic pressure. Aside from providing binary information about beat-to-beat changes in blood pressure, this system can also track median systolic, or diastolic, pressure levels from trial to trial by changing the constant pressure level in the cuff according to the percentage of K-sounds occurring during a given trial. For example, if 75% of heartbeats yield K-sounds, median systolic pressure is assumed to be greater than the cuff inflation pressure and the level set in the cuff is adjusted upward on the next trial, typically by 2 mm Hg. For low percentages (<25%), the cuff pressure is reduced by 2 mm Hg on the next trial. The constant-cuff method has been validated against intraarterial recording of blood pressure.

The second major approach to continuous assessment of blood pressure involves various tracking systems (Tursky, 1974). One recently developed system for systolic assessment is described. This system has a number of advantages, and it has been validated against intraarterial recordings of blood pressure (Shapiro, Greenstadt, Lane, & Rubinstein, 1981). Like the constant-cuff method, this tracking method employs a cuff and a procedure for detecting K-sounds. The cuff is initially inflated to the individual's clinically determined systolic blood pressure. Thereafter, the cuff pressure is increased or decreased by a given amount, depending on the presence or absence of a K-sound at each successive heartbeat. With the cuff pressure set at about systolic level, if a K-sound occurs, the subject's systolic blood pressure is higher than the cuff pressure, and the cuff pressure is increased by a given amount (2–3 mm Hg). Conversely, if a K-sound is absent, pressure in the cuff is decreased by the same amount. The cuff pressure change is made rapidly at a fixed time following the R-wave in the EKG. This beat-to-beat tracking of systolic blood pressure continues for the duration of the trial, and then the cuff is deflated. For the next trial, the cuff is initially inflated either to the last blood pressure value or to the mean blood pressure value of the previous trial, and tracking resumes. This tracking system can be recycled for as many trials as desired.

Both the constant-cuff and tracking-cuff systems described here can be used to provide beat-to-beat information about either systolic or diastolic pressure. The constant-cuff information is only binary in nature (above or below a given value), but the tracking-cuff information provides a closer estimation of absolute systolic (or diastolic) pressure.

The use of inexpensive electronic sphygmomanometers will likely play a growing role in behavioral studies, particularly those in which individuals are asked to record their own blood pressure for their own benefit or for other research purposes. (Self-monitoring and self-control procedures are described in Chapters 6 and 7.) Numerous devices are available commercially and are sold from various catalogs or even department stores. The critical feature concerns the reliability of the method for electronic detection of K-sounds. By and large, the devices are accurate and relatively efficient. Inasmuch as they provide a flash of light or brief tone for each detected K-sound, they are readily used by the average person and do not require the use of a stethoscope or lengthy training. Some current devices provide a digital (numerical) readout of systolic and diastolic pressure, and heart rate as well, thus requiring no subjective judgments whatsoever.

We have not dealt in any detail with such purported indirect measures of blood pressure or myocardial contractility as pulse transit time or carotid dp/dt because, in our opinion, complexly determined as they are by varying combinations of cardiac and vasomotor influences, they are more difficult to interpret compared to more direct measures of flow in the system or to indirect measures of blood pressure adapted from standard cuff techniques. (For further information on these alternative procedures see Light & Obrist, 1980; Obrist, Gaebelein, & Langer, 1975; Obrist, Light, McCubbin, & Hoffer, 1979.) The use of the pulse transit time measure in biofeedback research is also discussed in Chapters 4 and 6.

ANALYTIC ISSUES IN
CARDIOVASCULAR ASSESSMENT

From our earlier consideration of basic principles of cardiovascular physiology, it should now be clear that the most comprehensive approach to the analysis of changes in any given parameter of cardiovascular function must take into account two built-in characteristics of the cardiovascular system. First, parameters of cardiovascular function never exist as isolated phenomena but are highly interrelated with other aspects of the system's functioning. Second, there exists a wide array of mechanisms whereby information about change in one parameter of cardiovascular function influences both central nervous system (CNS) integrative mechanisms and other parameters, such that the status of the system and its components at any given point in time is going to play some role in the "change-ability" of any specific parameter whose response to some manipulation one wishes to measure.

The first characteristic means that, in order to understand what the cardiovascular system is "trying to accomplish" under any given set of experimental or real-life circumstances, it is necessary to employ multivariate techniques appropriate to the analysis of the integrated pattern of response of several parameters. For example, if one is measuring heart rate only and notes that a certain group of experimental subjects has a high heart rate, it will not be possible to determine on the basis of the heart rate data alone what the system is trying to accomplish. If, in addition, one measures FBF and finds that it is elevated, one could then begin to infer with more confidence that heart rate is elevated because the subjects are anxious or frightened by the experimental setting or manipulations employed, which is activating the defense reaction (see Chapter 3). On the other hand, if FBF is decreased, this inference would be untenable and one would then need to ask the subjects if they had recently eaten, since during active digestion there is an increased cardiac output, with vasodilatation in the mesenteric vascular bed and vasoconstriction in skeletal muscle. Without the information concerning important other aspects of cardiovascular system functioning, the heart rate information alone is difficult to interpret.

A variety of multivariate techniques is available for the analysis of patterned responses of interrelated parameters. For a detailed discussion of these techniques, the reader is referred to the excellent texts by Overall and Klett (1972) and Cohen and Cohen (1975). One example from our earlier work (Williams, Bittker, Buchsbaum, & Wynne, 1975) of the application of multivariate techniques to the discrimination of patterns of cardiovascular response has been commented upon by Hassett (1978). A principal-components analysis of changes in FBF, heart rate, systolic and diastolic blood pressure, and skin blood flow as indexed by digital pulse volume during a variety of experimental tasks showed that two patterns of response could account for most of the variance in response across all five parameters during the experimental conditions. The first component was positively weighted for increases in FBF, heart rate (HR), systolic blood pressure (SBP), and diastolic blood pressure (DBP) and negatively weighted for increased digital pulse amplitude. In other words, this component reflected a pattern of response in which FBF, HR, SBP, and DBP all increased while digital pulse amplitude decreased (the classical defense pattern as described in Chapter 3). The second component reflected a different pattern of response. It was negatively weighted for increase in FBF and HR but positively weighted for change in DBP. This represented a pattern in which FBF and HR *decreases* were observed in association with *increases* in DBP. As will be noted in Chapter 3, this represents the other pattern of cardiovascular response that we have described as occurring during sensory intake behavior.

Finally, it is necessary to consider the appropriate statistical approach to the measurement of changes in cardiovascular function. The simple difference (either in absolute terms or in terms of a percentage change score) between the value of a parameter before (pre) or after (post) some experimental manipulation is neither physiologically nor statistically valid. As already noted, physiologically it ignores the feedback and homeostatic mechanisms that tend to dampen changes in any given parameter under some conditions (e.g., baroreceptor reflex at rest) but not under others (e.g., baroreceptor reflex during the defense reaction). For a cogent discussion of why it is not statistically valid either, the reader is referred to Cohen and Cohen (1975), who also present one means of statistically dealing with the problems of measurement of change that is valid for physiological as well as other types of data of interest to the behavioral scientist. Briefly, this approach involves analysis of partial variance (APC) in which any relation between the pre and post values of the parameter in question is partialled out, such that the post-score becomes a measure of change in the parameter that is dependent only upon the intervening manipulation and independent of any relationship between the initial value and change in the parameter. This approach makes no assumption about the nature of the relationship between initial values and change scores; it empirically provides the investigator with a means of studying the effect of any experimental manipulation net of the prestimulus level of the parameter(s) of interest. Cohen and Cohen (1975) also deal with the multivariate generalization of this approach to the study of change.

While we have not attempted to be exhaustive in this chapter, we hope that the reader is sufficiently initiated into the complexities of the cardiovascular system to cope with the more substantive psychophysiological issues that we shall now address in Chapter 3.

REFERENCES

Brown, C. C. (Ed.). *Methods in psychophysiology.* Baltimore: Williams & Wilkins, 1967.
Cohen, J., & Cohen, P. *Applied multiple regression/correlation analysis for the behavioral sciences.* New York: Erlbaum, 1975.
Cook, M. R. Psychophysiology of peripheral vascular change. In P. A. Obrist, A. H. Black, J. Brener, & L. DiCara. (Eds.), *Cardiovascular psychophysiology.* Chicago: Aldine, 1974.
Folkow, B., & Neil, E. *Circulation.* New York: Oxford Univ. Press, 1971.

Hassett, J. *A primer of psychophysiology*. San Francisco: Freeman, 1978.

Jennings, J. R., Tahmaush, A. J., & Redmond, D. T. Non-invasive measurement of peripheral vascular activity. In I. Martin & P. H. Venables (Eds.), *Techniques in psychophysiology*. Chichester, England: Wiley, 1980.

Light, K. C., & Obrist, P. A. Cardiovascular response to stress: Effects of opportunity to avoid, shock experience, and performance feedback. *Psychophysiology*, 1980, *17*, 243–252.

Martin, I., & Venables, P. H. (Eds.). *Techniques in Psychophysiology*. Chichester, England: Wiley, 1980.

Obrist, P. A., Gaebelein, C. J., & Langer, A. W. Cardiovascular psychophysiology: Some contemporary methods of measurement. *American Psychologist*, 1975, *30*, 277–284.

Obrist, P. A., Light, K. C., McCubbin, J. A., & Hoffer, J. L. Pulse transit time: Relationship to blood pressure and myocardial performance. *Psychophysiology*, 1979, *16*, 292–306.

Overall, J. E., & Klett, C. J. *Applied multivariate analysis*. New York: McGraw-Hill, 1972.

Sarnoff, S. J., Mitchell, J. H., Gilmore, J. P., & Remensnyder, J. P. Homeometric autoregulation in the heart. *Circulation Research*, 1960, *8*, 1077.

Shapiro, D., Greenstadt, L., Lane, J. D., & Rubinstein, L. Tracking-cuff system for beat-to-beat recording of blood pressure. *Psychophysiology*, 1981, *18*, 129–136.

Stern, R. M., Ray, W. J., & Davis, C. M. *Psychophysiological recording*. New York: Oxford Univ., Press, 1980.

Thompson, R. F., & Patterson, M. M. (Eds.). *Biolectric recording techniques*. New York: Academic Press, 1974.

Tursky, B. The indirect recording of human blood pressure. In P. A. Obrist, A. H. Black, J. Brener, and L. V. DiCara (Eds.), *Cardiovascular psychophysiology*. Chicago: Aldine, 1974.

Tursky, B., Shapiro, D., & Schwartz, G. Automated constant-cuff pressure system to measure average systolic and diastolic pressure in man. IEEE *Transactions in Biomedical Engineering*, 1972, *19*, 271–276.

Whitney, R. J. The measurement of volume changes in human limits. *Journal of Physiology* (London), 1953, *121*, 1–27.

Williams, R. B., Bittker, F. E., Buchsbaum, M. S., & Wynne, L. C. Cardiovascular and neurophysiologic correlates of sensory intake and rejection: I. Effect of cognitive tasks. *Psychophysiology*, 1975, *12*, 427–432.

Venables, P. H., & Martin, I. *Manual of psychophysiological techniques*. Chichester, England: Wiley, 1967.

3

Introduction to Cardiovascular Psychophysiology

In Chapters 5 and 6 we shall discuss the role of behavioral factors in the etiology and pathogenesis of coronary heart disease and hypertension, as well as the use of behavioral approaches in the prevention, treatment, and rehabilitation of these major cardiovascular disorders. Insofar as environmental events and their impact upon the behavior of the organism are playing a role in the etiolgoy and pathogenesis of cardiovascular disease, it is self-evident that this role is mediated via the effects of organism–environment interactions upon physiological and neuroendocrine mechanisms that ordinarily serve to maintain cardiovascular homeostasis. Thus, an understanding of the role of behavioral factors in cardiovascular disease will depend ultimately upon our being able to define patterns of cardiovascular and neuroendocrine response that are reliably linked with specific patterns of behavioral adjustment to environmental demands. The study of such linkages—cardiovascular psychophysiology—is the subject of this chapter.

Historically, a model of the type, stress → disease, was to explain the role of behavioral factors in cardiovascular disease. Under this model, stress was nonspecific, leading to a general increase in arousal level (Duffy, 1962), with the eventful result that a disease process becomes initiated. Recent increases in our knowledge show that different organism–environment interactions are associated with qualitatively different patterns of cardiovascular response. Thus, it now appears possible to specify intervening psychophysiological mechanisms in much greater detail than was provided for in the nonspecific unidimensional arousal model.

The transduction of organism–environment interactions into patterns of cardiovascular and neuroendocrine response undoubtedly occurs in the brain. Previously, central nervous system (CNS) regulation of cardiovascular functions was understood in terms of various "centers," such as the medullary vasomotor center, where detailed studies (Alexander, 1946) mapped areas where electrical stimulation resulted in rises or falls in heart rate or blood pressure. Advances in the understanding of CNS regulation of cardiovascular function led Hilton to propose a modification of the earlier conceputalization that focused on brain-stem centers. He suggests

> that a new approach may be made by starting from the view that the central nervous system is organized to produce not single, isolated variables, but *integrated patterns* of response. Any variable which can be described or measured independently is actually a component of several such patterns.... In this system, the repertoire of patterned response [may be] very small [Hilton, 1975, 214; emphasis added].

Korner and Simon (1975) extend this reasoning by suggesting that the autonomic nervous system is set up to integrate "not only autonomic but also somatic and behavioral responses by which the organism meets the stressful requirements of real life [p. 339]." Thus, the older view that a given behavior "causes" an increase in blood pressure, for example, appears inconsistent with modern concepts of CNS regulation of cardiovascular function. The brain is organized to produce *both* somatomotor and cardiovascular "behaviors" as components of a single integrated pattern, depending upon the adjustments required by events. A number of such integrated patterns of response have now been identified in association with organism–environment interactions that lead to exercise, fight or flight, feeding, and diving. (See Abboud, Heistad, Mark, & Schmid, 1976 for a review.)

Among the "integrated patterns of responses" (Hilton, 1975) that have been studied, the best known and most extensively studied is that known as the defense reaction, consisting of intense affect, heightened somatomotor activity, increased cardiac output, and a shunting of blood from skin and viscera to the skeletal muscle vasculature. All these coordinated responses have been shown to be mediated by a common brain system (Abrahams, Hilton, & Zbrozyna, 1960), and several investigators (Abboud, 1976; Folkow & Neil, 1971; Henry, Ely, & Stephens, 1972) have proposed that the effects of repeated activations of the defense reaction upon baroreceptor function and vascular structure could be important in the pathogenesis of cardiovascular disease. It is important to consider whether there might be other integrated patterns of response, wherein the somatomotor, cardiovascular, and neuroendocrine components are qualitatively different from those observed during the defense reaction. Hallback (1976) has addressed this issue:

> It seems likely that the defense reaction, which so far is the best known of the emotionally induced behavioral responses, is only one of several patterns where central and peripheral neurohormonal adjustments, if often and powerfully elic-

ited, may produce serious disturbances both concerning organ function and mental state [p. 17].

It is perhaps not too surprising, therefore, that recent investigations have suggested that in addition to the defense reaction, wherein blood pressure elevations are achieved via increases in cardiac output, there appears to be another, qualitatively different response pattern, with blood pressure increasing in association with increased peripheral resistance rather than cardiac output. The motoric behavioral correlates of this pattern, rather than the heightened somatomotor activity observed with the defense reaction, appear to involve an actual diminution of somatomotor activity—often, it now appears, in the service of paying close attention to environmental stimuli.

Based upon the foregoing introduction, several premises can now be formulated to guide our thinking in the remainder of this chapter reviewing basic cardiovascular psychophysiology:

1. A given behavior does not directly "cause" a cardiovascular or neuroendocrine response. Rather, both the behavior and the cardiovascular and neuroendocrine responses are common components of an organized response pattern integrated by the CNS to meet the needs arising from a given organism–environment interaction.

2. It will be recognized that the use of the word *behavior* in the preceding paragraph refers to somatomotor activity. Actually, a more rational view that emerges from the stated premise is that an observable (i.e., measurable) alteration in any function of the organism in association with a given organism–environment interaction should be viewed as an aspect of the organism's behavior. Hence, not only somatomotor, but also physiological and neuroendocrine adjustments should be considered as making up the behavior of the organism.

3. The study of *single* responses (e.g., the blood pressure or heart rate response to any stimulus) can at best provide only an incomplete picture of basic cardiovascular psychophysiology in the intact functioning organism. This is because, as already noted, the organizing principle of organism adjustment to the environment involves shifting patterns of integrated somatomotor, physiological, and neuroendocrine behaviors that are appropriate to the given organism–environment interaction. Thus, a rational approach to cardiovascular psychophysiology will involve the determination of which patterns of somatomotor, physiological, and neuroendocrine response occur reliably in association with which types of organism–environment interactions.

We shall now review in some detail the experimental evidence establishing the existence of patterns of somatomotor, physiological, and neuroendocrine response in association with two types of organism–environment interactions.

One of these patterns is that known as the defense reaction, though, as will be noted, it also appears to occur in association with mental work. The other, which does not have nearly as long and venerable a history, appears to occur when the organism is engaged in attentive observation of the environment. It should be noted that, while the defense reaction pattern is well established and a standard feature in the "emotions" section of even basic physiology texts (e.g., Folkow & Neil, 1971), the second pattern and what Cohen and Obrist (1975) have termed the *adequate stimuli* for its elicitation remain to be fully understood, and differences of interpretation continue to abound. The view we present will, therefore, represent our interpretations of the available evidence; however, where this differs from the views of others, we shall attempt to consider alternative conceptualizations.

Finally, a word about organization. The two patterns of cardiovascular response upon which we shall focus in the remainder of this chapter are (*a*) pressor responses mediated largely by increased cardiac output; and (*b*) pressor responses mediated largely by increased total peripheral resistance. As noted earlier, whatever the nature of the specific environmental stimuli that are capable of activating these two response patterns, the site of transduction of such stimuli into the specific cardiovascular response patterns is surely the brain. Therefore, in each case we shall begin with a consideration of *brain mechanisms* known to mediate each of the two response patterns, along with somatomotor responses that have been observed in association with activation of those brain mechanisms. We shall next consider the evidence from both animal and human behavioral studies wherein various environmental manipulations have been employed to elicit a somatomotor response with observation of the concomitant physiological and neuroendocrine responses. We shall then present a model that synthesizes our thinking regarding the two response patterns. Finally, we shall address the issue of individual differences—a key concept for understanding why, despite identical environmental stimuli, some individuals will exhibit behavioral responses that differ in magnitude or even direction in comparison to others.

THE DEFENSE REACTION: INCREASED CARDIAC OUTPUT AND MUSCLE VASODILATATION

Brain Mechanisms

The key element in the cardiovascular response component of the defense reaction is a pressor response mediated by increased cardiac output, which is shunted into the skeletal muscle vascular bed. The CNS mediation of this response pattern has been amply documented.

Stimulation of points in the premotor cortex, the amygdala, the hypothalamus, the mesencephalic tegmentum, and the central gray matter of the anesthetized cat has been shown to result in marked increase in cardiac output; concomitantly, a vasoconstriction in the skin and viscera and an active vasodilatation in skeletal muscle is also observed (Abrahams *et al.*, 1960). The resultant blood pressure increase is due primarily to the increased cardiac output, since the total peripheral resistance response is variable, depending upon the relative magnitudes of the vasoconstrictor and vasodilator responses in skin–viscera and muscle, respectively. The vasoconstrictor effects are mediated peripherally by release of norepinephrine from sympathetic nerves innervating the skin and viscera. In contrast, the vasodilatation is mediated by release of acetylcholine from sympathetic nerves in muscle, as well as by stimulation of beta-receptors in muscle by epinephrine released from the adrenal medulla. While the presence of sympathetic cholinergic vasodilatation appears firmly established with regard to carnivores, there is some doubt about whether it occurs in primates (Schramm, Honig, & Bignall, 1971; Uvnas, 1966), where the principal mechanism would appear to involve beta-adrenergic stimulation. An important related effect of stimulation of brain areas giving rise to the increased output–muscle vasodilator response pattern is an attenuation of the baroreceptor-mediated inhibition of sympathetic outflow (Gebber & Snyder, 1970; Wenner-gren, Lisander, & Oberg, 1976). Thus, homeostatic mechanisms that would retard the pressor response are inhibited during brain stimulation, resulting in increased cardiac output and muscle vasodilatation.

Hess (1949) used the term *defense reaction* to describe a behavior pattern that can be elicited by stimulation of certain points in the hypothalamus of the conscious cat and that consists of an initial alerting followed by either flight or attack. Abrahams *et al.* (1960) showed that points in the anesthetized cat's brain where stimulation results in active vasodilatation in skeletal muscle, vasoconstriction in skin and viscera, and increase in cardiac output are also points where stimulation in the conscious animal results in coordinated defense behavior. They concluded that "regions of the hypothalamus, mensencephalic tegmentum, and gray matter function as reflex centers of the coordinated autonomic and behavioral responses that comprise the defense reaction [p. 509]."

Behavioral Studies

An extensive body of research led Brod (1970) to conclude that the cardiovascular response pattern associated with "defense" behavior in humans is identical in most respects to that seen in animals during stimulation of the hypothalamic defense area. A variety of experimental paradigms have been employed to elicit such behavior in humans, including mental arithmetic with harassment (Brod, Fencl, Hejl, & Jirka, 1959), leading subjects to believe that they have been accidently given a dangerous intravenous injection (Stead, Warren, Merrill, & Brannon, 1945), cardiac catheterization (Stead *et al.*, 1945), and the stress of an important medical school examination (Hickman, Cargill, & Golden, 1948). In each of these studies, both the emotional and cardiovascular response patterns observed appeared to correspond closely to that seen with hypothalamic stimulation in animals. While it might be tempting to conceptualize these findings as showing that the emergency behavioral response "caused" the increased cardiac output and muscle vasodilatation, we believe that a more correct interpretation is that the experimental procedures used in these studies activated the brain system responsible for mediating "the coordinated autonomic and behavioral responses that comprise the defense reaction [Abrahams *et al.*, 1960, p. 509]." This system appears to serve to prepare the organism for sudden, intense motor activity as would be required for fight or flight in the context of an environmental situation where there is perceived to be a threat to the organism's integrity.

In contrast to the situations described in the preceding paragraph, which place clear demands on the subjects to prepare for emergency motoric activity, other studies have employed less obviously threatening procedures, such as word association testing (Williams, Frankel, Gillin, & Weiss, 1973) and mental arithmetic without any harassment (Williams, Bittker, Buchsbaum, & Wynne, 1975), and found that the cardiovascular response pattern was qualitatively the same as in the "more stressful" situations—increased heart rate, muscle vasodilatation, and vasoconstriction in skin. The magnitude of response, however, was not as large. Such observations as these are consistent with the postulation by Lacey and Lacey (1974) that "mental work"—even with no overt requirements for increased motoric activity—can also activate the brain system responsible for integrating the cardiovascular response pattern seen during the defense reaction. Obrist (1976) has conceptualized those situations giving rise to a cardiac output pressor response as ones in which "active coping" is required of the organism in terms of motoric response. If this proves to be a correct interpretation, it would require a central mechanism whereby "mental" and "physical" work are somehow neurally linked. This is not a trivial issue, since it raises important questions concerning the adequate stimuli (Cohen & Obrist, 1975) for activating the CNS system that coordinates the expression of the defense reaction. If it does not require such extreme environmental situations as those clearly perceivable as emergencies, calling for immediate action, but can be activated by situations requiring such forms of mental work as performing mental arithmetic or remembering a telephone number, then the number of instances during the course of any ordinary day when the individual experiences an increased blood pressure with activation of the cardiac output–muscle vasodilatation pattern would be markedly increased.

The peripheral mechanisms accounting for the muscle vasodilatation observed during behavioral activation of the defense reaction involve both the release of epinephrine from the adrenal medulla (Lindgren, Rosen, & Uvnas, 1959) and activation of the sympathetic cholinergic vasodilator nerves (Uvnas, 1966). While the existence of the sympathetic cholinergic vasodilator input to muscles has been readily demonstrated in cats, dogs, and other carnivorous species, efforts have been unsuccessful in demonstrating this input in rodents and primates (Uvnas, 1966), raising doubt that such a neural input is present in humans. Attempts to identify the mechanisms underlying the skeletal muscle vasodilatation during elicitation of the defense reaction in humans have utilized beta-adrenergic blockade to assess the role of epinephrine released from the adrenal medulla and cholinergic blockade with atropine to assess the contribution of cholinergic vasodilator nerves (Barcroft, Brod, Hejl, Hirjarvi, & Kitchin, 1960). Although these studies generally provided some support for the operation in humans of both potential peripheral mechanisms, some exceptions were noted. Thus, some subjects showed as great a skeletal muscle vasodilatation after either atropinization or beta-adrenergic blockade as they did before pharmacologic intervention. This uncertaintly does not alter the essential observation that a key element of the defense reaction, in humans as well as lower animals, is an active vasodilatation in skeletal muscle.

In summary, pressor responses mediated by increased cardiac output can be elicited via stimulation of certain brain areas. Such stimulation does not produce the increased cardiac output as an isolated event, but rather as one component of a complex behavioral–physiological response pattern. Other components of this pattern include vasodilatation in skeletal muscle, vasoconstriction in skin and viscera, increased somatomotor activity, and emotional display characterized by fight or flight, depending upon the situation and the response repertoire available to the organism involved. The anatomic localization of the brain system responsible for integrating this response pattern has been established in extensive studies using animal models as described here. However, the central neurochemical substrate of this pattern remains to be elucidated. While it is clear that environmental situations calling for an emergency response to perceived threat will activate the brain system subserving the defense reaction, there is some evidence that situations that call for mental work without direct requirements for emergency motor activity also elicit this response pattern.

Thus far we have reviewed evidence supporting the concept that, under certain conditions of organism–environment interaction, there exists an integrative system within the CNS that coordinates expression of a pattern of somatomotor–cardiovascular–neurohumoral responses—the defense reaction— that are appropriate for that interaction. We shall now present evidence for the existence of another, qualitatively different somatomotor–cardiovascular– neurohumoral response pattern, a key element of which is increased peripheral resistance with vasoconstriction in skeletal muscle. As with our consideration of the evidence pertaining to the defense reaction, our review of this different response pattern will proceed from brain mechanisms mediating increased peripheral resistance to behavioral studies wherein certain somatomotor behaviors are found reliably linked with peripheral resistance–muscle vasoconstrictor cardiovascular response in animals and humans.

THE SENSORY PROCESSING REACTION: INCREASED PERIPHERAL RESISTANCE AND MUSCLE VASOCONSTRICTION

Brain Mechanisms

Increased blood pressure secondary to stimulation of the hypothalamic defense area is due primarily to an increase in cardiac output. (The total peripheral resistance response varies depending upon the relative vasodilatation in muscle and vasoconstriction in skin and viscera.) In contrast, there have been reports of other brain areas where various manipulations lead to a pressor response due primarily to an increase in total peripheral resistance, with cardiac output remaining unchanged or even decreasing. While the behavioral correlates of most of these manipulations have been subjected to much less study than those associated with defense area stimulation, certain preliminary observations have been reported that support the notion of a distinct brain system mediating increased peripheral resistance responses.

Folkow and Rubinstein (1966) reported that stimulation in the lateral hypothalamic area of anesthetized cats resulted in skeletal muscle vasoconstriction. Morpurgo (1968) stimulated anesthetized rats within .5 mm of the midline in the posterior hypothalamic area and observed a consistent large pressor response (80–100 mm Hg) accompanied by a marked decrease in heart rate (−80 bpm), suggesting that the pressor response was due to increased peripheral resistance rather than to a cardiac output response to stimulation. This interpretation was supported by the observation that the alpha blocking agent phentolamine attenuated the pressor response as well as the heart rate decrease.

Reis and Doba (1974) found in the rat that bilateral lesions of the areas receiving the primary afferent terminals of the baroreceptors in the region of the nucleus tractus solitari (NTS) are followed by an acute fulminating hypertension that leads to death secondary to congestive heart failure within 4–6 h. The hypertension thus caused appears to be due entirely to an increase in total peripheral resistance, since the heart rate is unchanged and the blood pressure increase is reduced by the alpha-adrenergic blocking agent phentolamine. Supracollicular areas of the brain are involved in mediating the hypertension after NTS lesions, since midcollicular decerebration will abolish the hypertension.

Thus, brain stimulation leading to increased cardiac output is associated with muscle *vasodilatation;* however, when the predominant result of brain manipulation is increased total peripheral resistance, there is a *vasoconstriction* not only in skin and viscera but in the skeletal musculature as well. It should be noted that cardiac output and peripheral resistance have not been measured directly in these studies, and further studies are needed to confirm the assumptions that have been made. In addition, it would appear that, whereas the baroreceptor inhibitory mechanism is attenuated during pressor episodes resulting from defense area stimulation, with stimulation of brain areas associated with increased peripheral resistance, the baroreceptor reflex remains active in reducing heart rate.

An additional contrast between the brain mechanisms mediating cardiac output responses compared to peripheral resistance responses is to be found in considering the neurotransmitters that appear to mediate these response patterns. While little is known concerning the central neurotransmitters involved in mediating the increased cardiac output and muscle vasodilatation in conjunction with defense area stimulation, there is much evidence that central monamine neurons are involved in mediating the increased sympathetic outflow responsible for the increased peripheral resistance observed in various experimental paradigms.

The pioneering work of the Swedish investigators Dahlstrom and Fuxe (1965) and Understedt (1971), utilizing both fluorescence histology and specific biochemical lesions of catecholamine neurons with 6-hydroxydopamine (6-OHDA) in the mapping of central monamine pathways, has spawned a burgeoning area of research aimed at determining the role of these systems in regulating a wide range of bodily functions. A comprehensive picture of cardiovascular psychophysiology will depend ultimately upon inclusion of these CNS monamine systems in our conceptual schemata. It now appears, for example, that the vasomotor center in the medulla oblongata utilizes both catecholaminergic (Ito & Schanberg, 1974) and serotonergic (Ito & Schanberg, 1972) mechanisms in the regulation of peripheral cardiovascular function. The NTS, the first relay station for baroreceptor afferent input, is richly innervated with noradrenergic terminals that appear to play a key role in the cardiovascular regulatory functions of the brain stem. DeJong (DeJong, Zandberg, & Bohus, 1975) performed microinjections of norepinephrine (NE) into the NTS and observed a decrease in blood pressure. In contrast, destruction of NE cell bodies and terminals in this area and the spinal cord by intercisternal 6-OHDA blocks the appearance of hypertension after bilateral NTS lesions (Reis & Doba, 1974). Thus, the NTS appear to have NE receptors that when stimulated reduce the sympathetic outflow, while other NE terminals, outside the NTS, appear important in maintaining the increased sympathetic outflow associated with destruction of inhibitory NE neurons in NTS hypertension. One site of these excitory NE neurons is in the spinal cord, where intercisternal 6-OHDA causes a marked depletion of NE terminals (Reis & Doba, 1974). It may be recalled that midcollicular decerebration also reduces blood pressure in NTS hypertension. The massive sympathetic discharge associated with bilateral carotid occlusion (BCO) is likely mediated by the same mechanism that determines the increased sympathetic outflow in NTS hypertension. It is interesting, therefore, that the pressor response to BCO is reduced by perfusion of the caudal brain stem with alpha-adrenergic blocking agents and that this attenuation of the BCO pressor response by central alpha-adrenergic blockage is prevented by midcollicular decerebration (Tadepalli, Mills, & Schanberg, 1977). One possible site for the supracollicular NE receptors responsible for the increased sympathetic outflow in association with either BCO or NTS hypertension is suggested by the finding that the pressor response and associated heart rate decrease after posterior hypothalamic stimulation is blocked by destruction with 6-OHDA of NE terminals in that area (Przuntek, Guimaraes, & Phillippu, 1971).

Underlying the floor of the fourth ventricle is the locus coeruleus, a small bilateral collection of cell bodies that supplies all the noradrenergic terminals for the cerebral cortex, the cerebellum, and parts of the hypothalamus (Ungerstedt, 1971). Stimulation of the locus coeruleus was found to produce an increase in blood pressure that was blocked by lesions in the posterior hypothalamus (Przuntek & Phillippu, 1971). Thus, there is reason to believe that the noradrenergic terminals responsible for the increased sympathetic vasoconstrictor discharge resulting from posterior hypothalamic stimulation (Przuntek *et al.*, 1971) may have their origin in the locus coeruleus. It has been proposed (Ward & Gunn, 1976a,b) on the basis of observed cardiovascular responses to locus coeruleus stimulation that this collection of noradrenergic cell bodies plays a role in mediating autonomically caused cardiovascular responses to arousal and activation. In addition, the locus coeruleus appears involved in the regulation of sympathetic vasoconstrictor outflow in humans. Black and Petito (1976) report a 50-fold decrease in tyrosine hydroxylase (the rate-limiting enzyme in catecholamine synthesis) in the locus coeruleus of patients with idiopathic orthostatic hypotension in comparison to controls studied at autopsy.

While the final synthesis of the diverse findings reviewed here must await more definitive investigations, we believe that such evidence serves to document the hypothesis that, in addition to the increased cardiac output and muscle vasodilatation observed in association with stimulation of the defense areas of the brain, there exists a different CNS system that mediates an increase in peripheral resistance with an associated muscle vasoconstriction. Moreover, it appears that this CNS system mediating increased peripheral resistance–muscle vasoconstriction responses utilizes NE as a neurotransmitter, with the locus coeruleus and the posterior hypothalamic area being probable loci of the relevant noradrenergic neurons. Such a hypothesis is in accord with Haeusler's (1975) proposal that there are two noradrenergic systems in the brain concerned with regulation of sympathetic outflow to the vasculature. One, involving the posterior hypothalamus and possibly extending to the spinal cord, appears to mediate increased sympathetic vasoconstrictor outflow, while the other, centered in the NTS, appears involved in inhibition of sympathetic outflow. Undoubtedly, these mechanisms will ultimately need to be incorporated in any explanation of how certain types of organism–environment interaction are transduced into peripheral resistance–muscle vasoconstriction patterns of cardiovascular response.

We have reviewed here the data describing the behavioral effects (Abrahams *et al.*, 1960) of stimulation of those brain areas in which stimulation in the anesthetized animal produces the increase in cardiac output and muscle vasodilatation characteristic of the defense reaction. In contrast, there are no such systematic studies regarding the behavioral correlates of stimulation of those brain areas involved in mediating increased peripheral resistance and skeletal muscle vasoconstriction. Folkow and Rubinstein (1966) observed feeding behavior in response to stimulation of those lateral hypothalamic points where stimulation in the anesthetized cat caused muscle vasoconstriction. Morpurgo (1968) stimulated in chronic rats those posterior hypothalamic points associated with pressor-deceleratory responses in the anesthetized rat and observed "exploratory activity" initially, with a flight reaction ensuing with continued stimulation.

Such studies are only suggestive of the possible somatomotor behavioral component(s) of an integrated response pattern with a cardiovascular component of increased peripheral resistance and muscle vasoconstriction. In contrast to the absence of studies of behavioral response to brain stimulation productive of increased peripheral resistance and muscle vasoconstriction, there are a number of behavioral studies in which experimental manipulation of behavioral response requirements have been reported to cause a pressor response due to increased peripheral resistance and muscle vasoconstriction rather than increased cardiac output with muscle vasodilatation. A consideration of somatomotor behaviors observed in association with such peripheral resistance increases provides important clues regarding the behavioral correlates of activation of the brain system mediating increased peripheral resistance and muscle vasoconstriction.

Behavioral Studies

Zanchetti and co-workers (Adams, Baccelli, Mancia, & Zanchetti, 1971) observed the cardiovascular hemodynamics of the cat during both confrontation and fighting with another cat that was made aggressive by stimulation of the hypothalamic defense area. During actual fighting, or flight from the stimulated cat, the hemodynamically monitored cats exhibited the expected increased cardiac output and shunting of blood from skin and viscera to the vasodilated skeletal muscle vasculature. During *preparation for fighting*, however, both the observable behavior and monitored physiological responses were qualitatively different from those seen during fight or flight. During preparation, the cat "simply flinched, retracted its ears, dilated the pupils and *watched the attack cat closely* [Adams *et al.,* 1971, p. 329; emphasis added]." In marked contrast to the increased somatomotor activity and cardiac output with skeletal muscle vasodilatation observed during fight or flight, during preparation (i.e., while watching the other cat "closely") a low level of electromyographic (EMG) activity, a decrease in heart rate and cardiac output, and a *vasoconstriction* in the artery supplying the hind limb muscles were observed. On the basis of these observations, Zanchetti concludes that there appears to be a dual cardiovascular response pattern subserving emotional behavior—"one type being the usual companion of immobile confrontation of the preparatory stage, the other type being characteristic of emotional movement (the classical 'defense pattern') [Zanchetti, 1976, p. 421]."

Anderson and Brady (1971, 1972; Anderson & Tosheff, 1973) have studied the hemodynamic responses of dogs during preavoidance periods and during periods where bar pressing behavior was required to avoid painful electric shocks (see Figure 3.1). During avoidance periods, with the threat of shock and the frequent motoric activity to avoid the shock, they observed an increase in blood pressure that was mediated by an increase in cardiac output. In contrast, during the preavoidance hour, they observed "progressive decreases in cardiac output accompanied by decreases in both stroke volume and heart rate . . . concurrently [with] progressive elevations in arterial blood pressure . . . indicating progressive increases in total peripheral resistance [Anderson & Tosheff, 1973, p. 652]." In these studies, they did not specifically measure muscle hemodynamics. They interpret these findings as indicative of an alpha-adrenergic stimulation of a vasoconstrictive response that is partly accounted for by increased release of NE from the sympathetic nerves. The peripheral resistance-mediated pressor response during preavoidance occurs "under conditions of minimal activity in anticipation of an environment of imminent danger [Anderson & Tosheff, 1973, p. 653]." Anderson (Note 1) agrees with our suggestion that the dog's attentive observation of the shock-avoidance manipulanda is a cardinal feature of this "anticipation."

Grignolo and Williams (Note 2) report the occurrence of a phasic increase in blood pressure and decrease in heart rate during learned anticipation of painful footshocks in the rat. This hemodynamic pattern was interpreted as likely representing an increase in peripheral resistance. The behavior of the rats might best be described as "immobile anticipation" of the imminent footshock. Interestingly, the magnitude of the phasic pressor response was significantly attenuated by depletion of brain catecholamines by intercisternal injection of

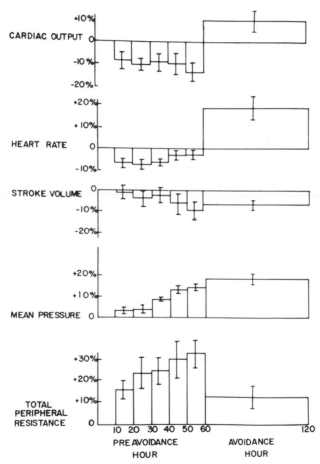

FIGURE 3.1. Average levels of cardiac output, heart rate, stroke volume, mean arterial pressure, and total peripheral resistance over successive 10 min intervals. [From D. E. Anderson, & J. G. Tosheff. Cardiac output and total peripheral resistance changes during preavoidance in the dog. *Journal of Applied Physiology,* 1973, 34, 652.]

6-OHDA 1 week before testing, while the heart rate decrease was unaffected. It may be speculated that such CNS catecholamine depletion reduced this sympathetically mediated pressor effect via action upon the locus coeruleus and/or posterior hypothalamic noradreneregic system involved in regulating sympathetic outflow as described previously (Przuntek & Phillippu, 1971).

Williams and Eichelman (1971) observed a significant decrease in blood pressure after shock-induced fighting in the rat. When two animals receive footshocks of much reduced intensity, the fighting behavior does not occur, but the significant blood pressure decrease after a series of 50 shocks delivered over 7 min is, if anything, enhanced. This blood pressure decrease appears to be reflexively induced in response to a sympathetic nerve-mediated pressor response during footshock, since the decrease is reversed to significant increase by pretreatment to destroy peripheral sympathetic nerves with intravenous 6-OHDA, but not by adrenalectomy (Williams, Eichelman, & Ng, 1979). Further studies showed that pretreatment to destroy CNS catecholamine neurons with intracisternal 6-OHDA also reversed the significant blood pressure decrease to a significant increase after footshock of rat pairs (Williams, Eichelman, & Ng, 1972). This finding provides another example of the possible involvement of CNS catecholamine systems in mediating an increased sympathetic vasoconstrictor outflow in association with a specific behavioral response. In the most recent study of this series, it was found that bilateral locus coeruleus lesions also reverse the blood pressure decrease after footshock of rat pairs (Williams, Richardson, & Eichelman, 1978), suggesting the involvement of the postulated locus coeruleus–posterior hypothalamic noradrenergic system in mediating this effect.

We interpret the studies cited as suggesting that the cardiovascular response of increased peripheral resistance (with muscle vasoconstriction) does indeed occur in association with specific types of behavioral responses. Whereas the increased cardiac output and muscle vasodilatation pattern occurs in association with either emergency fight–flight behavior or mental work, the behaviors that appear centrally integrated in association with increased peripheral resistance and muscle vasoconstriction have a quite different quality: "immobile confrontation" (Adams et al., 1971), "preavoidance" (Anderson & Tosheff, 1973, immobile anticipation (Grignolo & Williams, Note 2). A final conclusion regarding the precise nature of the behavioral correlates of increased peripheral resistance and muscle vasoconstriction is not possible on the basis of the animal studies cited here. The evidence available thus far does appear to warrant the conclusion that these behaviors are distinct from those observed in association with increased cardiac output and muscle vasodilatation.

A number of investigations utilizing human subjects provide further clues regarding the specific nature of the somatomotor behavioral response occurring in association with increased peripheral resistance and muscle vasoconstriction.

As noted earlier, the cardiovascular response pattern observed in association with experimental tasks requiring mental work (e.g., mental arithmetic) in humans consists of an increase in heart rate (and cardiac output) (Brod *et al.*, 1959; Lacey & Lacey, 1974), an increase in somatomotor activity (Brod *et al.*, 1959; Obrist, 1976), and a vasodilatation in skeletal muscle (Brod *et al.*, 1959; Williams *et al.*, 1975). Even though this pattern is reliably seen even when the experimental subjects are not led to believe that an emergency exists, we believe that activation of the brain's defense system provides an adequate explanation of the linkage between the behavior of mental work and the elaboration of the observed physiological response pattern.

The Laceys (Lacey, 1972; Lacey & Lacey, 1974) made the initial observations suggesting the existence of another behavioral–physiological response pattern qualitatively different from the so-called defense pattern. They found that stimulus conditions requiring mental work were associated with an increase in heart rate, as would be expected with activation of the defense system. In contrast, when the experimental conditions employed required the subjects to note and detect incoming (sensory) stimuli, the heart rate response was a deceleration—even though such other indexes of sympathetic nervous function as skin potential and pupillary diameter showed an activation pattern (Libby, Lacey, & Lacey, 1973). They termed this divergence of heart rate and other indexes of sympathetic function *directional fractionation*. As the subsequent review will suggest, this phenomenon of directional fractionation can be understood as part of another centrally integrated behavioral–physiological response pattern, which Williams (1981) has termed the *sensory intake reaction*.

The most extensively studied example of cardiac deceleration during sensory intake behavior is the beat-by-beat decrease in heart rate (often seen after an initial acceleration) that is observed with the approach of the imperative stimulus in the foreperiod of the standard reaction time task (Lacey & Lacey, 1974; Nowlin, Thompson, & Eisdorfer, 1969; Obrist, 1963). In addition, numerous studies have demonstrated sustained (tonic) heart rate decreases in association with sustained motivated attention to external sensory stimuli (Hare, Wood, Britain, & Shadman, 1970; Israel, 1969; Lewis, Kagan, Campbell, & Kalafat, 1966; Nowlin *et al.*, 1969). Of particular importance was a study by Coles (1972) in which he found the cardiac deceleratory response to be greater during a hard than during an easy sensory intake task. Traditional arousal theory (Duffy, 1962) would predict that the harder the task, the greater the physiological arousal and, hence, the higher the heart rate should be. The Laceys' suggestion that arousal may not be a unitary phenomenon, but that there may be different patterns of arousal (Lacey, 1967) depending upon whether the behavior observed can be characterized as sensory rejection (i.e., mental work) or sensory intake, would account for Coles's findings. This suggestion of the Laceys' is also quite consistent with the position outlined in the introduction to this chapter—that somatomotor behavior and physiological response are linked via activation of CNS systems that coordinate the expression of a (limited) number of behavioral–physiological response patterns.

In addition to having made the observation that the specific heart rate response during sensory intake is one of deceleration, the Laceys have also advanced hypothesis to answer the question "Why does the heart rate decelerate during attention and accelerate during motivated inattention?" (Lacey & Lacey, 1974). It is their position (the "afferent feedback hypothesis") that the heart rate deceleration during sensory intake is instrumental in facilitating sensory intake behavior. They cite evidence from the neurophysiological literature that suggests that increasing heart rate and blood pressure, by stimulating baroreceptors in the carotid sinus and aortic arch, can actually produce "a number of *inhibitory* effects on brain function and behavior [Lacey, 1972, p. 178]." Thus, the decreased baroreceptor discharge resulting from cardiac deceleration—the most effective stimulus to the baroreceptors is the rate of pressure change, dp/dt (Folkow & Neil, 1971)—could facilitate sensory intake by virtue of a reduction in the inhibition of brain function by baroreceptor input. The status of the afferent feedback hypothesis remains to be settled, as witnessed by criticisms of it (Elliott, 1972) and responses by the Laceys (Lacey & Lacey, 1974). An additional question concerns the effect of the *increased* dp/dt, which must surely occur during mental work, upon performance of tasks involving mental work: Would not the "inhibitory effects on brain function" (Lacey, 1972) of such an increase in dp/dt, and the resultant increase in baroreceptor discharge, impair mental work performance? The ultimate fate of the afferent feedback hypothesis does not alter the fact that the heart rate response observed in association with sensory intake behavior is qualitatively different from that during mental work. Nor does it alter the implications of that fact for understanding behavioral–cardiovascular interaction.

Another investigator who has addressed the issue of sensory intake behavior and its physiological correlates has been Obrist, who has called especial attention to the role of somatomotor activity as the most important variable for understanding physiological response during sensory intake beahvioral studies. In an extensive series of investigations, studying phasic heart rate changes in the classical aversive conditioning paradigm and the signaled reaction time task (see Obrist, 1976, for a review), Obrist and co-workers have confirmed the existence of the cardiac deceleratory response during the foreperiod of the reaction time task but also noted a concomitant, time-locked decrease in various indexes of somatomotor activity, including chin EMG, eye blinks, and gross body movements monitored by sensitive sensors attached to the subject's chair.

Obrist has concluded, presumably on the basis of his findings that heart rate and somatomotor response appear to occur together, that knowledge of the heart rate response is redundant in terms of implications for behavior. That is, Obrist believes that heart rate may be a useful tool *only* to the extent that it provides an index of the activity of the striate musculature (Obrist, 1976). This conclusion seems unwarranted on two grounds. First, this emphasis on which single variable is "best" misses the point that it is the *pattern* of physiological responses that provides the most comprehensive knowledge regarding how the brain is acting to integrate the behavioral and physiological responses. Second, it is far more likely that knowledge concerning the cardiovascular rather than the somatomotor components, will increase our understanding of the role of behavior in the pathogenesis of cardiovascular disease.

A third line of investigation relevant to the issue of the specific nature of the eliciting stimuli and somatomotor behavior that may be associated with increased peripheral resistance cardiovascular responses has been conducted by Williams and co-workers. An initial study (McKegney & Williams, 1967; Williams & McKegney, 1965) of 10 normotensive and 13 hypertensive inpatients showed that diastolic blood pressure was significantly elevated during a discussion of personally relevant topics among both groups. A subsequent study was undertaken to identify the key aspect of the behavior during the interview that induced the diastolic pressor response. It was found among 9 inpatients and 8 normal volunteers that a diastolic pressure increase during an interview similar to that of the first study was related more to the process of interpersonal interaction than to the novelty of the interview or its personal content (Williams, Kimball, & Willard, 1973). When there was relatively little interpersonal interaction, the diastolic pressor increase during the interview averaged only 3 mm Hg, whereas during interviews with relatively more interpersonal interaction, but similar content, an average diastolic pressor response of 6 mm Hg was observed. These findings were interpreted as being in substantial agreement with earlier work (see Singer, 1974, for a review), suggesting that the level of "engagement-involvement" with one's current surroundings is a key determinant of cardiovascular responsivity during various experimental conditions.

In a subsequent study (Bittker, Buchsbaum, Williams, & Wynne, 1975; Williams *et al.*, 1975), an attempt was made to identify more specifically those aspects of behavior occurring during interpersonal interaction that are relevant for specific *patterns* of cardiovascular response, rather than for the isolated single variable of diastolic blood pressure. Nineteen normal volunteers were subjected to experimental conditions requiring sensory intake behavior (word identification task), mental work without attention to external stimuli (mental arithmetic), and interpersonal interaction (interview) with concurrent monitoring of five cardiovascular response parameters—systolic blood pressure (BP), diastolic blood pressure, forearm blood flow (FBF), digital pulse amplitude, and heart rate. In addition, the interview was observed and the degree of "attentiveness to the interviewer" was independently rated. The patterns of cardiovascular response during each attentional condition were significantly dif-

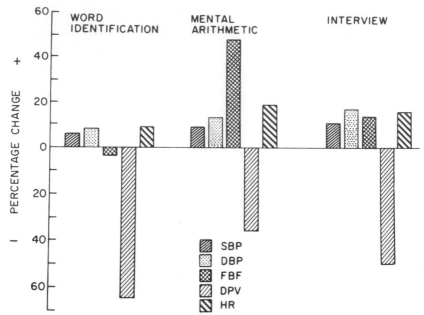

FIGURE 3.2. Changes in five cardiovascular parameters during work identification, mental arithmetic, and interview. [From R. B. Williams, T. E. Bittker, M. S. Buchsbaum, & L. C. Wynne. Cardiovascular and neurophysiological correlates of sensory intake and rejection: I. Effect of cognitive tasks. *Psychophysiology*, 1975, *12*, 429.]

ferent from prior baselines and from each other (see Figure 3.2). Further analysis of the data revealed that a derived measure of forearm vasomotor tone, forearm vascular resistance (mean BP/FBF), *increased* significantly during the word identification task but *decreased* significantly during mental arithmetic (see Figure 3.3).

Multivariate analysis of the data from this study showed FBF to be the strongest variable in differentiating the psychological response to the three experimental conditions. Principal-components analysis of cardiovascular response scores during the three conditions showed two independent components that accounted for about ¾ of the variance in cardiovascular response. In one component, *increases* in FBF were found positively correlated with increased systolic and diastolic blood pressure and heart rate, whereas in the second component, *decreases* in FBF were correlated with diastolic blood pressure increases and heart rate decreases. On the basis of these findings, it was concluded that the cardiovascular response during sensory intake behaivor is more complex than a simple passive decrease in heart rate, but rather is characterized by "a specific pattern of active cardiovascular response, a cardinal feature of which is a vasoconstriction of skeletal muscle [Williams *et al.*, 1975, p. 429]."

The findings (Bittker *et al.*, 1975) relating to cardiovascular response during the interview segment of this study were in accord with those during the other two attentional conditions. Whereas during the word identification and mental arithmetic tasks the attentional demands were uniformly applied across all subjects, the interview represented a more naturalistic situation in which individual attentional preferences might be more freely expressed. Accordingly, it was found that the 10 subjects who were rated as more attentive to the interviewer during the interview exhibited a higher baseline forearm vascular resistance (FVR) level than the 9 nonattenders and showed a significant increase from the initial FVR level during the interview; in contrast, the nonattenders

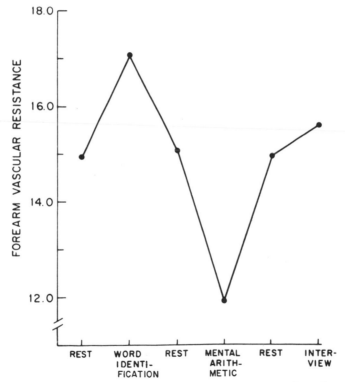

FIGURE 3.3. Forearm vascular resistance (FVR) response to sensory intake and mental work tasks. [From R. B. Williams, T. E. Bittker, M. S. Buchsbaum, & L. C. Wynne. Cardiovascular and neurophysiological correlates of sensory intake and rejection: I. Effect of cognitive tasks. *Psychophysiology*, 1975, *12*, 429.]

showed a significant decrease during the interview (see Figure 3.4). Thus, the more naturalistically occurring behavior of being attentive to another person was associated with a forearm vasomotor response like that exhibited during a sensory intake task, whereas the behavior of not being attentive to the interviewer (but to one's own thoughts and associations?) was associated with a forearm vasomotor response like that exhibited during a mental work task. This suggests that where the individual can engage in a freer range of behaviors during a given situation, the cardiovascular and somatomotor behaviors continue to pattern together as they do when the situational demands are more explicit for either sensory intake or mental work (Hassett, 1979).

To determine the role of the sympathetic nervous system in mediating the hemodynamic responses observed in the forearm during tasks requiring sensory intake as compared to mental work, an additional study was carried out subjecting 22 normal volunteers to a task requiring continuous monitoring of visual stimuli (Continuous Performance Task—CPT) and to a task requiring mental work (mental arithmetic without demands for sensory processing) (Williams, Buchsbaum, Henry, & Wooten, Note 3). The sympathetic response during these tasks and preceding baselines are assayed in terms of total plasma catecholamine levels in blood samples withdrawn via an indwelling intravenous needle during the last minute of each 5-min segment. The FBF responses to the two tasks were significantly different, with a small decrease during the CPT and a large increase during mental arithmetic. The difference between the plasma catecholamine increases during the CPT and mental arithmetic nar-

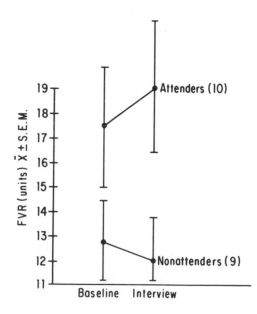

FIGURE 3.4. Forearm vascular resistance (FVR) response to an interview.

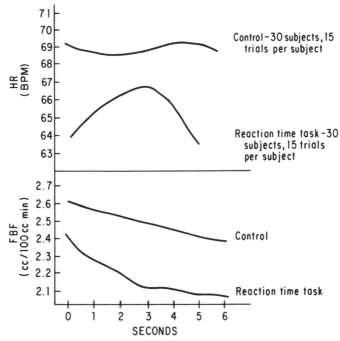

FIGURE 3.5. Phasic forearm blood flow (FBF) and heart rate (HR) during control period and reaction time tasks.

rowly missed significance by a two-tailed t test. These findings suggest that an activation of the sympathetic nervous system is involved in mediating the cardiovascular response during sensory intake behavior.

In another study, Williams, Bauknight, Cleveland, and Jackson (Note 4) investigated not only tonic but phasic forearm hemodynamic responses during the foreperiod of the standard reaction time task. Thirty-one young normal volunteers were monitored in terms of second-by-second FBF and heart rate levels during a baseline period in which no stimuli were presented. Following this, they performed in the signaled reaction time task, with a warning signal followed in 6 sec by a response signal to which they pressed a key. In the reaction time portion of the study, the warning and response signals were timed to occur concomitantly with the FBF determinations, which were done over a 10-sec interval using venous occlusion strain gauge plethysmography (Whitney, 1953). Highly reliable differences, in terms of both tonic levels and phasic changes during the foreperiod, were observed between the FBF and heart rate responses during the control period and those during the foreperiod of the reaction time task (see Figure 3.5).

In terms of tonic levels of heart rate and FBF, the imposition of the warning signal and response contingency was associated with significant decreases in both FBF and heart rate averaged across the 6-sec foreperiod compared to the comparable interval during the control condition, when no warning or response contingencies were present. Were it not for earlier data (Bittker et al., 1975; Williams et al., 1975) showing an active increase in FVR during sensory intake behavior, it would be reasonable to interpret the observed decreases in heart rate and FBF as reflective of a decreased arousal. The earlier hemodynamic data suggest, however, that the cardiovascular response during sensory intake is an active one. Furthermore, it is difficult to conceive that the behavioral state of sitting with one's eyes peering into the eyepiece of a tachistoscope with instructions to pay close attention and "press the key as quickly as possible when the respond signal comes on" could possibly be less "arousing" than the state of sitting quietly with instructions "to just sit and count slowly from 1 to 100 while we take some baseline measures."

Further evidence that the forearm vasomotor response observed in this study was an active one is provided by consideration of the phasic heart rate and FBF responses (see Figure 3.5). There was a sharp fall in FBF during the first 3 sec of the reaction time foreperiod; the significant quadratic trend confirmed the reliability of this phenomenon. Under the control condition, no such quadratic trend was present. At the same time the FBF was falling, however, a sharp increase was observed in heart rate, again highly reliable as reflected in the significant quadratic trend.

Thus, with a theoretical model in which only the increased FBF and heart rate of the defense reaction are viewed as reflecting increased arousal, it would be hard to explan the diverging heart rate and FBF responses during the first half of the foreperiod. On the other hand, a model that also includes a skeletal muscle vasoconstriction as a potential arousal pattern would better account for the observed results. The data also suggest that the cardiac deceleratory response, beginning at the 3-sec mark, when the FBF fall is leveling off, could be a result of activation of baroreceptor reflex mechanisms.

Obrist and co-workers (Obrist, Lawler, Howard, Smithson, Martin, & Manning, 1974) observed an increase in diastolic blood pressure, measured intraarterially, in humans during the foreperiod of the reaction time task. They interpreted this diastolic pressure response as the result either of an increase in peripheral resistance or of the increase in heart rate that they also observed early in the foreperiod before the deceleratory phase later in the foreperiod. More recently, Obrist advanced the view (Obrist, 1976) that the diastolic pressor response of the earlier study (Obrist et al., 1974) is mediated by an increased peripheral resistance, despite the absence of any direct evidence relating to systematic or local vascular resistance levels. The evidence of increased FVR during a sensory intake task (Williams et al., 1975), and attentive regard of the interviewer during an interview (Bittker *et al.*, 1975), along with the divergence of FBF or heart rate responses during the early part of the foreperiod of the reaction time task (Williams *et al.*, 1975) do, however, constitute more direct evidence of a peripheral vasoconstrictor-mediated increase in resistance to flow.

A PROPOSED MODEL

A question that now arises concerns the nature of the somatomotor behavior that is associated with the peripheral resistance response pattern. If such a cardiovascular response pattern does deserve consideration along with the defense reaction pattern as one of the basic response patterns, what constitutes an "adequate stimulus" (Cohen & Obrist, 1975) for eliciting it? Although by no means conclusive, the animal literature cited earlier suggested consideration of behavioral states ranging from "immobile confrontation" (Zanchetti, 1976) to footshock of rat pairs (Williams & Eichelman, 1971). The human studies we have reviewed here suggest to us that motivated intention to note and detect incoming (sensory) stimuli (Lacey & Lacey, 1974) is also characteristic of those states in association with which muscle vasoconstrictor responses are observed. Obrist (1976) has proposed the terms *active coping* and *passive coping* to describe the essential elements of those behavioral states in which cardiac output and peripheral resistance response patterns are observed, respectively. It may well be that these two views are not mutually exclusive but focus on different aspects of the organism's behavior as relevant correlates of cardiovascular response patterning. Certainly, the process of sensory intake is readily characterizable as "passive" in that it requires a receptive orientation on the part of the organism. We are of the opinion, however, that it is the *intention* to engage in sensory intake, rather than the diminution of somatomotor acitvity, that is the essential determinant of whether a sympathetically mediated generalized vasoconstrictor response occurs. Furthermore, this intention is also seen as determining the decreased somatomotor activity. This view is consistent with that of Zanchetti, who proposed dual cardiovascular response patterns occurring in association with emotional behavior, the first involving the increased cardiac output and muscle vasodilatation characteristic of emotional movement (the classical defense pattern) and the second involving the vasoconstriction in skeletal muscle observed during "immobile confrontation" (Zanchetti, 1976). Another problem with the concept of active coping, which Obrist proposes as the behavioral correlate of the increased cardiac output response pattern, is seen upon consideration that mental work, such as mental arithmetic, is also associated with the cardiac output–muscle vasodilatation pattern. It would appear necessary to postulate some neurophysiological connection between mental and physical work, with the exercise system outflow to the cardiovascular system also being activated in association with mental work.

While the resolution of the issues raised in the preceding discussion will require further investigation, we shall summarize the evidence that has been reviewed thus far by presenting a model that represents Williams's (1981) synthesis of the available evidence relating to behavioral–cardiovascular patterning. Extensive research is needed to evaluate this model, to characterize its various components, and, eventually, to apply it toward identification of the basic mechanisms whereby behavioral factors play a role in the pathogenesis of cardiovascular disease. This model does not necessarily represent final truth; it is presented here as a means of organizing a wide range of empirical findings and as a heuristic guide for planning the needed research.

As illustrated in Figure 3.6, an incoming novel stimulus results in alerting, or orienting, on the part of the organism. It should be noted here that there is an extensive literature relating to what has been termed the *orienting reflex* (see Sokolow, 1963, for a review). This reflex consists of phasic responses of a number of physiological parameters following a stimulus. Such responses show decrement with repeated presentations of the given stimulus, or habituation. As will become evident from the following discussion, we are not concerned with the orienting reflex but with those behavioral and physiological events that occur later, following cognitive appraisal.

The process of cognitive appraisal involves an evaluation of the characteristics of the stimulus and the formulation of a decision regarding the import of the stimulus for the organism. As depicted in Figure 3.6, that decision could lead to one of two major types of outcome. On the one hand, it could lead to emotional motor or mental work. Where danger is perceived, and fight or flight is required, this would represent an activation of the classical defense pattern (Zanchetti, 1976). Where the decision results in mental work (e.g., mental arithmetic or trying to remember some past data, such as a telephone number), a similar qualitative, but perhaps quantitatively less intense, activation of the same pattern of physiological responses ensues. On the other hand, when the decision that emerges from the process of cognitive appraisal is that the stimulus has interest and more information about it is desirable, the organism maintains an ongoing orientation of the relevant sense organs toward that stimulus, and the pattern of physiological responses depicted in Figure 3.6 under "Sensory Intake" is observed.

A number of factors play a role in determining the outcome of the process of cognitive appraisal. First, the qualitites of the stimulus and the context in which it occurs are important in determining the decision that is made. For example, a growling tiger seen in the setting of a zoo, behind the stout bars of its cage, would be likely to arouse interest and hence continued sensory intake

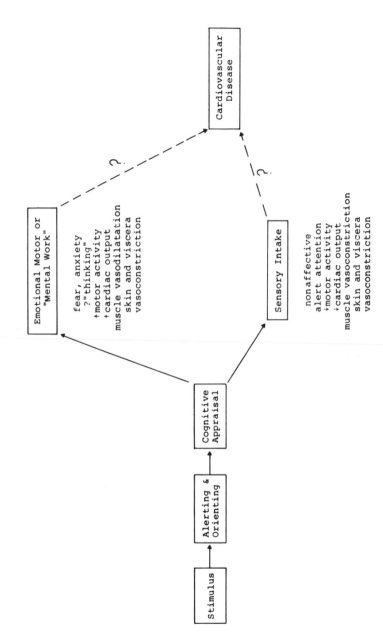

FIGURE 3.6. Theoretical model: Emotional motor or mental work and sensory intake response patterns.

after the initial orienting and cognitive appraisal. On the other hand, the same stimulus encountered on a narrow jungle path in the wilds of northcentral India would be far more likely to lead to a decision that danger exists, and an entirely different pattern of physiological responses would ensue. A second source of variance in determining the outcome of the cognitive appraisal process involves the past experience and certain characteristics of the organism that encounters the stimulus. An illustration of this is the increase in blood pressure mediated by increased peripheral resistance observed in dogs during a pre-avoidance hour (Anderson & Brady, 1971, 1972; Anderson & Tosheff, 1973). This pattern of physiological response was not observed during the first pre-avoidance hours but only after the past experience of the animals could be inferred to have brought about a learning process such that the stimulus parameters reliably led to the decision that the avoidance period would follow shortly. Another source of individual differences in decision outcomes is to be found in the area of enduring characteristics of the individual, or cognitive styles, to be considered later.

The evidence reviewed thus far leads to postulation of two basic patterns of physiological responses that reliably occur in association with specific behavioral states (Cohen & Obrist, 1975). One of these patterns, depicted in Figure 3.6 under "Emotional Motor or Mental Work," consists of increased motor activity and cardiac output, with vasodilatation in skeletal muscle and vasoconstriction in the skin and viscera. This pattern is widely known and enjoys general acceptance as the defense reaction. The other pattern, depicted under "Sensory Intake," is not so well established. Our postulation of its existence as one of the basic response patterns is based upon eivdence from a wide variety of experimental studies employing both animals and humans as subjects. Clearly, extensive further research will be required to establish the validity of this hypothesized physiological response pattern as occurring in association with sensory intake behavior and to characterize the peripheral neural mechanisms mediating its expression.

It is worthwhile at this point to consider how the brain might translate the decision emerging from the process of cognitive appraisal into the efferent pattern necessary to bring about the physiological responses characteristic of either the established defense pattern or the hypothesized sensory intake pattern. With regard to the defense pattern, it is well established (Abrahams *et al.*, 1960) that stimulation of any of a number of points within the hypothalamic defense area brings about the complete behavioral–physiological response pattern depicted under "Emotional Motor or Mental Work" in Figure 3.6. The process of cognitive appraisal undoubtedly involves cortical processes. There are known pathways whereby cortical stimulation can result in activation of the hypothalamic defense area (Abrahams *et al.*, 1960). Thus, it appears highly likely that, instead of activation by stimulating electrode, another potential activating mechanism of the hypothalamic defense area would be via descending cortical inputs that could be activated as a result of those processes involved in cognitive appraisal. The reliable occurrence of the defense pattern of physiological response in humans subjected to experimental paradigms that presumably elicit fear has been cited (Brod, 1970) as evidence for such a mechanism.

With regard to the sensory intake pattern, the anatomic distribution of the CNS integration system mediating its expression remains to be identified. The confirmation of the reliable occurrence of a behavioral–cardiovascular response pattern like that depicted under "Sensory Intake" in Figure 3.6 would constitute evidence that such an integration system does indeed exist. Earlier, we reviewed evidence suggests that sympathetic vasoconstrictor outflow to the muscle vasculature is mediated by noradrenergic neurons in the CNS and that the locus coeruleus and the posterior hypothalamic area are CNS areas where the relevant noradrenergic neurons may be localized. Furthermore, evidence was reviewed suggesting the mediation of behaviorally induced sympathetic vasoconstrictor responses by CNS noradrenergic neurons.

Such evidence, while by no means conclusive, does suggest that it is a CNS system employing NE as a transmitter that serves to mediate the expression of those cardiovascular responses observed during sensory intake. As with the defense pattern, this system would presumably be activated via descending pathways from the cortex upon the appropriate outcome of the cognitive appraisal process.

Thus far we have dealt mainly with the somatomotor and physiological components of response patterns observed in association with various organism–environment interactions. Data pertaining to the possible neurohumoral components of the two patterns we have described are inconclusive at present. One reason for this may be that heretofore the defense pattern was the only response pattern recognized, and thus, the experimental conditions employed did not take into account the possibility of other patterns of response. This problem is revealed by the scattered findings that a variety of neuroendocrine substances in blood have been reported to increase in response to "stress," but there has been much confusion regarding what constitutes an adequate stimulus (stress) for a given neuroendocrine response.

Mason (1975) has noted that "striking changes in levels of many hormones, including cortisol, epinephrine, growth hormone, prolactin, thyroxine, insulin, and testosterone often occur . . . in response to stressful stimuli [p. 8]." Most often the stresses have been of the type that would suggest that the defense system has been activated. However, there has been some evidence that different organism–environment interactions are associated with different patterns of hormonal response. For example, for a cortisol response to occur, it appears necessary for the organism to experience emotional distress as a result of a given environmental event, suggesting a defense reaction mechanism. Mason (1968) has suggested further that plasma epinephrine increases in situations where novelty and uncertainty surround the presentation of aversive stimuli; in contrast, when the conditions are familiar and stereotyped, only an increase in NE levels is observed. Mandler (1967) has proposed that when relevant behavioral responses are unavailable to the organism, a predominant release of epinephrine occurs, whereas NE release predominates when relevant behavior is available for meeting the requirements of the situation. Thus, cortisol and both epinephrine and NE would be expected to increase with activation of the defense system, whereas only NE would be expected to increase during sensory processing. Although incomplete as yet, studies in progress in our laboratory tend to support this prediction (Williams, Kuhn, Lane, Schanberg, White, & Melosh, Note 5).

The primary focus thus far has been on the characterization of patterns of cardiovascular response that appear reliably in association with specific patterns of behavioral adjustment. We believe that it would be useful, however, to see if the different patterns of cardiovascular response that can be identified are also reliably accompanied by distinct patterns of neuroendocrine response. Evidence of different patterns of neuroendocrine response in association with the two proposed cardiovascular response patterns would provide further evidence of the distinctiveness of the cardiovascular patterns, would suggest peripheral mechanisms for their mediation, and would provide further clues as to the involvement of CNS monoamine systems in their mediation.

It was proposed some time ago that situations in which the subject's predominant affect is one of anger are associated with a pattern of physiological response like that produced by the action of NE, whereas an epinephrine-like response is seen in situations inducing fear or anxiety (Ax, 1953; Funkenstein, King, & Drolette, 1954; Schachter, 1957). The absence of adequate assays for these hormones in blood at the time made it impossible to confirm this hypothesis, and no evidence has been forthcoming in recent years that is supportive. It may be, however, that the two patterns of cardiovascular response that we have proposed here could account for the two different physiological response patterns observed in those early studies. Fear or anxiety would be likely to activate the defense system, with its beta-adrenergic response pattern of increased cardiac output and muscle vasodilatation. On the other hand, a subject responding to the same situation with anger might be expected to be more vigilant, to be more engaged in sensory intake to appraise the situation, rather than preparing to flee. If so, then activation of the sensory intake response pattern with its muscle vasoconstriction and stable or declining cardiac output could provide an explanation for the mechanism underlying the different physiological response during anger. The advent of more sensitive assays for blood levels of NE and epinephrine (Passon & Peuler, 1973) and their application in studying the neuroendocrine correlates of the different cardiovascular patterns we have postulated could help to understand both the specific sympathetic mediation of the patterns we postulate and the older findings relating to fear and anger.

THE ROLE OF INDIVIDUAL DIFFERENCES

Thus far we have focused upon the uniformity of physiological response patterns of groups of individuals exposed to the same experimental conditions. It is a fact of life, however, that there are wide variations in the responses observed that become evident upon examination of the range of individuals who make up a given experimental sample. These individual differences can be categorized in terms of either psychological or physiological factors. A brief review of some of the evidence pertaining to individual differences in cardiovascular responses will serve to support our hypothesis of two different basic cardiovascular response patterns and to indicate the need to control for such differences in studies of behavioral–cardiovascular interactions.

A wide variety of psychological characteristics of individuals have been found to correlate with cardiovascular response during various behavioral paradigms. These characteristics might be described as "cognitive styles"— enduring strategies that the individual employs in dealing with the stimuli of his or her external environment. Subjects whose average cortical evoked potential pattern to lights of increasing intensity indicates a preference on their part to attend to environmental stimuli when given free choice exhibit significantly higher levels of FVR under "no instruction" conditions than do subjects with evoked potential patterns suggestive of a tendency not to attend to environmental stimuli (Williams et al., 1975). Levelers and sharpeners differ with regard to their tendency to pay close attention to the details of environmental stimuli, with sharpeners characteristically preferring to be more attentive to external details. Israel (1969) found that sharpeners showed more frequent and larger cardiac decelerations in anticipation of affectual visual stimuli in comparison to levelers. Subjects with an internal locus of control are described as being more alert to those aspects of the environment which provide useful information for future behavior [Rotter, 1966]. Williams, Poon, and Burdette (1977) found 15 subjects with internal locus of control to show a more pronounced muscle vasoconstrictor response during a visual monitoring task when compared to 14 subjects with external locus of control. Dronsejko (1972) found that field-independent subjects show a greater cardiac deceleration in anticipation of an impending sensory event when compared to field-dependent subjects. She interpreted this finding as resulting from a greater level of "attentive observation" in anticipation of the stimulus on the part of field-independent subjects. Eysenck (1967) emphasized the importance of enduring tendencies to attend to the external world of sensory stimuli (extraversion) versus the inner world of thoughts and ideas (introversion) as one of the two main dimensions of personality.

In addition to the individual differences with regard to cognitive style, it also appears likely that individual differences in cardiovascular response during varying organism–environment interactions are also related to measurable differences in sympathetic nervous function.

The demonstrations that the soluble fraction of dopamine-beta-hydroxylase (DBH: EC 1.14.2.1), located in synaptic vesicles of sympathetic neurons, is released concomitantly with NE (Viveros, Arqueros, Arqueros, & Kirshner, 1968) and that large amounts of the enzyme accumulate in serum (Weinshilboum & Axelrod, 1971) led to the suggestion that serum DBH concentrations might serve as an accurate index of sympathetic nervous system activity. Evi-

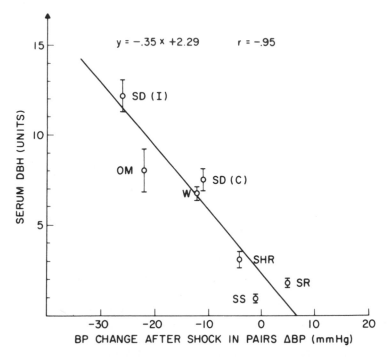

FIGURE 3.7. Serum dopamine-beta-hydroxylase (DBH) levels and blood pressure (BP) changes after shock in rat pairs. [From F. Lamprecht, B. S. Eichelman, R. B. Williams, G. F. Wooten, & I. J. Kopin. Serum dopamine-beta-hydroxylase (DBH) activity and blood pressure response of rat strains to shock-induced fighting. *Psychosomatic Medicine,* 1974, *36, 300.*]

dence is also accumulating that alterations in serum DBH have been reported to occur in experimental animals exposed to immobilization (Lamprecht, Williams, & Kopin, 1973), chronic swim stress (Roffman, Freedman, & Goldstein, 1973), and sympathetic stimulation following baroreceptor denervation (Ngai, Dairman, Marchelle, & Spector, 1974) and in human quadriplegic patients during sympathetically mediated hypertensive crisis (Naftchi, Wooten, Towman, & Axelrod, 1973). A number of clinical studies have reported increased levels of serum DBH among patients with hypertension (Geffen, Rush, Louis, & Doyle, 1973; Horowitz, Alexander, Lovenberg, & Keiser, 1973; Stone, Gunnells, Robinson, Schanberg & Kirshner, 1974; Wetterberg, Aberg, & Ross, 1972). However, others failed to detect "any alteration" of serum DBH activity in a large group of patients with hypertension (Horowitz *et al.*, 1973).

Evidence that serum DBH levels provide potentially useful information regarding a characteristic of the organism is provided by the finding that the characteristic DBH level in the blood of various rat strains is related to the blood pressure response to shock-induced fighting. As shown in Figure 3.7, those rat strains with high serum DBH levels, whether on a genetic basis or on the basis of immobilization stress (SD[I]), exhibit a larger blood pressure fall after shock-induced fighting than do strains with low DBH levels (Lamprecht, Eichelman, Williams, Wooten, & Kopin, 1974). Since the blood pressure fall after shock-induced fighting requires the integrity of peripheral sympathetic nerves (Williams *et al.*, 1979), we have concluded that it is the result of a reflex depressor response following activation of these nerves during fighting. Thus, these findings also support the hypothesis that characteristic levels of peripheral sympathetic nerve activity, as reflected in serum DBH levels, are an important determinant of cardiovascular response during certain types of organism–environment interactions.

SUMMARY

The brain is organized to integrate coordinated patterns of somatomotor, physiological, and neuroendocrine behavioral response that are appropriate adjustments to the requirements of specific types of organism–environment interactions. Therefore, a rational approach to the field of cardiovascular psychophysiology would attempt to define those patterns of somatomotor, cardiovascular, and neuroendocrine response that are found to be reliably linked in association with specific types of organism–environment interactions. As illustrated in Figure 3.6, one such reliable pattern is that known as the defense reaction (emotional motor or mental work), consisting of (*a*) intense affect or cognitive elaboration, (*b*) increased somatomotor activity, (*c*) increased cardiac output, (*d*) muscle vasodilatation, and (*e*) vasoconstriction elsewhere. Although the CNS neurotransmitter substrate mediating this reaction is not known, the anatomic distribution of sites where stimulation elicits the full-blown defense reaction has been extensively defined. In addition to the defense reaction pattern, we have described another, qualitatively different pattern of somatomotor, cardiovascular, and neuroendocrine response that we have termed the *sensory intake reaction,* consisting of (*a*) relatively little affect but alert attentive observation, (*b*) a diminution in somatomotor activity, (*c*) decreased, or at least unincreased, cardiac output, and (*d*) vasoconstriction in muscle as well as skin and viscera. There is preliminary evidence that CNS mediation of this sensory processing reaction involves noradrenergic neurons located within a circuit involving the locus coeruleus and the posterior hypothalamic area.

While further research may help to refine our understanding of the adequate stimuli for eliciting each of these reactions, we believe that the basic cardiovascular components of the two patterns will ultimately be shown to be as we have described them here: (*a*) a pressor response mediated primarily by increased cardiac output, with that increased output being shunted away from skin and viscera to muscle, and (*b*) a pressor response mediated primarily by a generalized vasoconstriction in muscle as well as skin and viscera, with cardiac output decreasing or showing no change. Furthermore, as we will detail in Chapters 5 and 6, it is likely that, to the extent behavioral influences are playing a role in the etiology and pathogenesis of cardiovascular disease, it will be via the mediation of these two basic response patterns.

REFERENCE NOTES

1. Anderson, D. E. Personal communication, October 1977.
2. Grignolo, A., & Williams, R. B. *Anticipatory cardiovascular responses to footshock: Mediation by brain amines.* Paper presented at the annual meeting of the Society for Psychophysiological Research, Salt Lake City, October 1974.
3. Williams, R. B., Buchsbaum, M. S., Henry, D., & Wooten, G. F. *Peripheral sympathetic nerve activity and sensory intake behavior: A newly recognized association.* Paper presented at the annual meeting of the American Psychosomatic Society, Philadelphia, March 1974.
4. Williams, R. B., Bauknight, T., Cleveland, W., & Jackson, M. S. *Phasic forearm blood flow responses during the preparatory interval of a reaction time task.* Paper presented at the annual meeting of the Society for Psychophysiological Research, Salt Lake City, October 1979.
5. Williams, R. B., Kuhn, C., Lane, J. D., Schanberg, S. M., White, A., & Melosh, W. *Patterns of neuroendocrine response during two types of mental problem solving.* Paper presented at the annual meeting of the American College of Neuropsychopharmacology, San Juan, December 1980.

REFERENCES

Abboud, F. M. Relaxation, autonomic control and hypertension. *New England Journal of Medicine*, 1976, *294*, 107–109.

Abboud, F., Heistad, D. D., Mark, A. L., & Schmid, P. G. Reflex control of the peripheral circulation. *Progress in Cardiovascular Diseases*, 1976, *18*, 371–402.

Abrahams, V. C., Hilton, S. M., & Zbrozyna, A. Active muscle vasodilatation produced by stimulation of the brain stem: Its significance in the defense reaction. *Journal of Physiology* (London), 1960, *154*, 491–513.

Adams, D. B., Baccelli, G., Mancia, G., & Zanchetti, A. Relation of cardiovascular changes in fighting to emotion and exercise. *Journal of Physiology* (London), 1971, *212*, 321–335.

Alexander, R. S. Tonic and reflex functions of medullary sympathetic cardiovascular centers. *Journal of Neurophysiology*, 1946, *9*, 205–217.

Anderson, D. E., & Brady, J. B. Preavoidance blood pressure elevations accompanied by heart rate decreases in the dog. *Science*, 1971, *172*, 595–597.

Anderson, D. E., & Brady, J. B. Differential preparatory cardiovascular responses to aversive and appetitive behavioral conditioning. *Conditional Reflex*, 1972, 82–96.

Anderson, D. E., & Tosheff, J. G. Cardiac output and total peripheral resistance changes during preavoidance in the dog. *Journal of Applied Physiology*, 1973, *34*, 650–654.

Ax, A. F. The physiological differentiation between fear and anger in humans. *Psychosomatic Medicine*, 1953, *15*, 432–442.

Barcroft, H., Brod, J., Hejl, Z., Hirjarvi, E. A. & Kitchin, A. H. The mechanism of the vasodilatation in the forearm muscle during stress (mental arithmetic). *Clinical Science*, 1960, *19*, 577–586.

Bittker, T. E., Buchsbaum, M. S., Williams, R. B., & Wynne, L. C. Cardiovascular and neurophysiologic correlates of sensory intake and rejection: II. Interview behavior. *Psychophysiology*, 1975, *12*, 434–438.

Black, I. B., & Petito, C. K. Catecholamine enzymes in the degenerative neurological disease idiopathic orthostatic hypotension. *Science*, 1976, *192*, 910–912.

Brod, J. Haemodynamics and emotional stress. In M. Koster, H. Musaph, & P. Visser (Eds.), *Psychosomatics in essential hypertension*. New York: Prager, 1970.

Brod, J., Fencl, V. S., Hejl, Z., & Jirka, J. Circulatory changes underlying blood pressure elevation during acute emotional stress (mental arithmetic) in normotensive and hypertensive subjects. *Clinical Science*, 1959, *18*, 269–279.

Cohen, D. H., & Obrist, P. A. Interactions between behavior and the cardiovascular system. *Circulation Research*, 1975, *37*, 693–701.

Coles, M. G. H. Cardiac and respiratory activity during visual search. *Journal of Experimental Psychology*, 1972, *96*, 371–379.

Dahlstrom, A., & Fuxe, K. Evidence for the existence of monoamine neurones in the central nervous system. *Acta Physiologica Scandinavia*, 1965, *64*, (Suppl. No. 274), 1–36.

DeJong, W., Zandberg, P., & Bohus, B. Central inhibitory noradrenergic cardiovascular control. *Progress in Brain Research*, 1975, *42*, 285–298.

Dronsejko, K. Effects of CS duration and instructional set on cardiac anticipatory responses to stress in field dependent and independent subjects. *Psychophysiology*, 1972, *9*, 1–13.

Duffy, E. *Activation and behavior*. New York: Wiley, 1962.

Elliott, R. The significance of heart rate for behavior: A critique of Lacey's hypothesis. *Journal of Personality and Social Psychology*, 1972, *22*, 398–409.

Eysenck, H. J., *The biological basis of personality*. Springfield, Ill.: Thomas, 1967.

Folkow, B., & Neil, E. *Circulation*. New York: Oxford University Press, 1971.

Folkow, B., & Rubinstein, E. H. The functional role of some autonomic and behavioral patterns evoked from the lateral hypothalamus of the cat. *Acta Physiologica Scandinavia*, 1966, *66*, 182–188.

Funkenstein, D. H., King, S. H., & Drolette, M. A. The direction of anger during a laboratory stress-inducing situation. *Psychosomatic Medicine*, 1954, *16*, 404–413.

Gebber, G. L., & Snyder, D. W. Hypothalamic control of baroreceptor reflexes. *American Journal of Physiology*, 1970, *218*, 124–131.

Geffen, L. B., Rush, R. A., Louis, W. J., & Doyle, A. E. Plasma dopamine-hydroxylase and noradrenaline amounts in essential hypertension. *Clinical Science*, 1973, *44*, 617–620.

Haeusler, G. Cardiovascular regulation by central adrenergic mechanisms and its alteration by hypotensive drugs. *Circulation Research*, 1975, 36 & 37, (Suppl. No. 1), 1–223.

Hallback, M. Autonomic adjustments in situations of mental stress. *Advances in Clinical Pharmacology*, 1976, *12*, 14–20.

Hare, R., Wood, K., Britain, S., & Shadman, J. Autonomic response to affective visual stimulation. *Psychophysiology* 1970, *7*, 408–417.

Hassett, J. *A primer of psychophysiology*. San Francisco: Freeman, 1979

Henry, J. P., Ely, D. L., & Stephens, P. M. Mental factors and cardiovascular disease. *Psychiatric Annals*, 1972, *2*, 25–46.

Hess, W. R. *Das Zwischenhern*. Basel, Verlag: Schwade and Co., 1949.

Hickman, J. B., Cargill, W. H., & Golden, A. Cardiovascular reactions to emotional stimuli. Effect on the cardiac output, arteriovenous oxygen difference, arterial pressure, and peripheral resistance. *Journal of Clinical Investigation*, 1948, *27*, 290–298.

Hilton, S. M. Ways of viewing the central nervous control of the circulation—old and new. *Brain Research*, 1975, *87*, 213–219.

Horowitz, D., Alexander, R. W., Lovenberg, W., & Keiser, H. R. Human serum dopamine-hydroxylase. Relationship to hypertension and sympathetic activity. *Circulation*, 1973, *32*, 594–599.

Israel, N. R. Leveling–sharpening and anticipatory cardiac responses. *Psychosomatic Medicine*, 1969, *31*, 499–509.

Ito, A., & Schanberg, S. M. Central nervous system mechanisms responsible for blood pressure induced by P-chlorophenylalanine. *Journal of Pharmacology and Experimental Therapeutics*, 1972, *181*, 65–74.

Ito, A., & Schanberg, S. M. Maintenance of tonic vasomotor activity in alpha and beta adrenergic mechanisms in medullary cardiovascular centers. *Journal of Pharmacology and Experimental Therapeutics*, 1974, *189*, 392–404.

Korner, P. I., & Simon, E. Comments on session III—regional organization of autonomic nervous system. *Brain Research*, 1975, *87*, 339–340.

Lacey, J. I. Somatic response patterning and stress: Some revisions of activation theory. In M. H. Appley & R. Turnbull (Eds.), *Psychological stress: issues in research*. New York: Appleton, 1967.

Lacey, J. I. Some cardiovascular correlates of sensorimotor behavior: Examples of visceral afferent feedback. In C. H. Hockman (Ed.), *Limbic system mechanisms and autonomic functioning*. Springfield, Ill.: Thomas, 1972.

Lacey, J. I., & Lacey, B. C. On heart rate responses and behavior: A reply to Elliott. *Journal of Personality and Social Psychology*, 1974, *30*, 1–18.

Lamprecht, F., Eichelman, B. S., Williams, R. B., Wooten, G. F., & Kopin, I. J. Serum dopamine-beta-hydroxylase (DBH) activity in blood pressure response of rat strains to shock-induced fighting. *Psychosomatic Medicine*, 1974, *36*, 298–303.

Lamprecht, F., Williams, R. B., & Kopin, I. J. Serum dopamine-beta-hydroxylase during development of immobilization-induced hypertension. *Endocrinology*, 1973, *92*, 953–956.

44

Lewis, M., Kagan, J., Campbell, H., & Kalafat, J. The cardiac response as a correlate of attention in infants. *Child Development,* 1966, 37, 63–71.

Libby, W. L., Lacey, B. C., & Lacey, J. I. Pupillary and cardiac activity during visual attention. *Psychophysiology,* 1973, 10, 270–294.

Lindgren, P., Rosen, A., & Uvnas, B. The release of catechols from the adrenal medulla on activation of the bulbar part of the sympathetic vasodilator outflow in cats. *Acta Physiologica Scandinavia,* 1959, 47, 233–242.

McKegney, F. P., & Williams, R. B. Psychological aspects of hypertension: II. The differential influence of interview variables on blood pressure. *American Journal of Psychiatry,* 1967, 123, 1539–1543.

Mandler, G. The conditions for emotional behavior. In D. C. Glass (Ed.), *Neurophysiology and emotion.* New York: Russell Sage Foundation, 1967.

Mason, J. W. Organization of the multiple endocrine responses to advoidance in the monkey. *Psychosomatic Medicine,* 1968, 30, 774–790.

Mason, J. W. A historical view of the stress field. *Journal of Human Stress,* 1975, 1, 6–12.

Morpurgo, E. Pharmacological modifications of sympathetic responses elicited by hypothalamic stimulation in the rat. *British Journal of Pharmacology,* 1968, 34, 532–542.

Naftchi, N. E., Wooten, G. F., Towman, E. M., & Axelrod, J. Concomitant changes in dopamine-p-hydroxylase (DPH) activity and hemodynamics during hypertensive crisis in quad-replegia. *Federation Proceedings,* 1973, 32, 708.

Ngai, S. H., Dairman, W., Marchell, M., & Spector, S. Dopamine-beta-hydroxylase in dog lymph—effect of sympathetic activation. *Life Sciences,* 1974, 14 (21) 2431–2439.

Nowlin, J. B., Thompson, L. W., & Eisdorfer, C. Cardiovascular response to reaction time performance. *Psychophysiology,* 1969, 5, 568. (Abstract)

Obrist, P. A. Cardiovascular differentiation of sensory stimuli. *Psychosomatic Medicine,* 1963, 25, 450–459.

Obrist, P. A. The cardiovascular–behavioral interaction—as it appears today. *Psychophysiology,* 1976, 13, 95–107.

Obrist, P. A., Lawler, J. E., Howard, J. L., Smithson, K. W., Martin, P. L., & Manning, J. Sympathetic influences on the heart in humans: Effects on contractility and heart rate of acute stress. *Psychophysiology,* 1974, 11, 405–527.

Passon, P. G., & Peuler, J. D. A simplified radiometric assay for plasma norepinephrine and epinephrine. *Analytical Biochemistry,* 1973, 51, 618.

Przuntek, H., Guimaraes, S., & Phillippu, A. Importance of adrenergic neurons of the brain for the rise of blood pressure evoked by hypothalamic stimulation. *Naunyn Schmiedebergs. Archive fur Pharmakologie* (Berlin), 1971, 271, 311–319.

Przuntek, H., & Phillippu, A. Reduced pressor responses to stimulation of the locus coeruleus after lesion of posterior hypothalamus. *Naunyn Schmiedebergs. Archive fur Pharmakologie* (Berlin), 1973, 276, 119–122.

Reis, D. J., & Doba, N. The central nervous system and neurogenic hypertension. *Progress in Cardiovascular Disease,* 1974, 17, 51–71.

Roffman, M., Freedman, L. S., & Goldstein, M. The effects of acute and chronic swim stress on dopamine-p-hydroxylase activity. *Life Science,* 1973, 12, 369–376.

Rotter, J. B. Generalized expectancies for internal versus external control of reinforcement. *Psychology Monographs,* 1966, 80 (1, Whole No. 609).

Schachter, J. Pain, fear and anger in hypertensives and normotensives. *Psychosomatic Medicine,* 1957, 19, 17–29.

Schramm, L. P., Honig, B. R., & Bignall, K. E. Active muscle vasodilatation in primates homolo-
gous with sympathetic vasodilatation in carnivores. *American Journal of Physiology*, 1971, *221*,
768–777.

Singer, M. T. Engagement-involvement: A central phenomenon in psychophysiological research.
Psychosomatic Medicine, 1974, *36*, 1–17.

Sokolow, Y. N. *Perception and the conditioned reflex*. New York: Pergamon, 1963.

Stead, E. A., Warren, J. V., Merrill, A. J., & Brannon, E. S. The cardiac output in male subjects
as measured by the technique of right atrial catherization. Normal values with observations on
the effect of anxiety and tilting. *Journal of Clinical Investigation*, 1945, *24*, 290–298.

Stone, R. A., Gunnells, J. C., Robinson, R. R., Schanberg, S. M., & Kirshner, N. Dopamine-
beta-hydroxylase in primary and secondary hypertension. *Circulation Research*, 1974, *34*, & 35
(Suppl. 1), 47–56.

Tadepalli, A. S., Mills, E., & Schanberg, S. M. Central depression of carotid baroreceptor pressor
response, arterial pressure and heart rate by 5-hydroxytroptopahn: Influence of supra-collicular
areas of the brain. *Journal of Pharmacology and Experimental Therapeutics*, 1977, *202*, 310–319.

Understedt, U. Stereotaxic mapping of the monoamine pathways in the rat brain. *Acta Physiologica
Scandinavia*, 1971, *367*, 1–48.

Uvnas, B. Cholinergic vasodilator nerves. *Federation Proceedings*, 1966, *25*, 1618–1622.

Viveros, O. H., Arqueros, O. H., Arqueros, L., & Kirshner, N. Quantal secretion from adrenal
medulla: All-or-none release of storage vesicle content. *Science*, 1969, *165*, 911–913.

Ward, D. G., & Gunn, C. G. Locus coeruleus complex: Differential modulation of depressor
mechanisms. *Brain Research*, 1976, *107*, 407–411. (a)

Ward, D. G., & Gunn C. G. Locus coeruleus complex: Elicitation of a pressor response and a brain
stem region necessary for its occurrence. *Brain Research*, 1976, *107*, 401–406. (b)

Weinshilboum, R. M., & Axelrod, J. Serum dopamine-beta-hydroxylase activity. *Circulation Research*, 1971, *28*, 307–315.

Wennergren, G., Lisander, B., & Oberg, B. Interaction between the hypothalamic defense reaction and cardiac ventricular receptor reflexes. *Acta Physiologica Scandanavia*, 1976, *96*, 532–
547.

Wetterberg, L., Aberg, H., & Ross, S. B. Plasma dopamine-beta-hydroxylase activity in hypertension and various neuropsychiatric disorders. *Scandinavian Journal of Clinical Laboratory Investigation*, 1972, *30*, 283–289.

Whitney, R. J. The measurement of volume changes in human limbs. *Journal of Physiology* (London) 1953, *121*, 1–27.

Williams, R. B. Behavioral factors in cardiovascular disease: An update. In J. W. Hurst (Ed.),
Update V: The Heart. New York: McGraw-Hill, 1981, 219–230.

Williams, R. B., Bittker, T. E., Buchsbaum, M. S., & Wynne, L. C. Cardiovascular and
neurophysiologic correlates of sensory intake and rejection: I. Effect of cognitive tasks. *Psychophysiology*, 1975, *12*, 427–432.

Williams, R. B., & Eichelman, B. S. Social setting: Influence upon physiological response to
electric shock in the rat. *Science*, 1971, *174*, 613–614.

Williams, R. B., Eichelman, B. S., & Ng, L. K. Y. Brain amine depletion reverses the blood
pressure response to footshock in the rat. *Nature (New Biology)*, 1972, *240*, 276–277.

Williams, R. B., Eichelman, B. S., & Ng, L. K. Y. Behavioral determinants of the patterned
sympathetic nervous system activation mediating the blood pressure response to electric shock
in the rat. *Psychophysiology*, 1979, *16*, 89–93.

Williams, R. B., Frankel, B. L. Gillin, J. C., & Weiss, J. Cardiovascular response during a word
association test and an interview. *Psychophysiology*, 1973, *10*, 571–577.

Williams, R. B., Kimball, C. P., & Willard, H. N. The influence of interpersonal interaction upon
diastolic blood pressure. *Psychosomatic Medicine*, 1973, *34*, 194–198.

Williams, R. B., & McKegney, F. P. Psychological aspects of hypertension: I. The influence of experimental interview variables on blood pressure. *Yale Journal of Biology and Medicine,* 1965, *38,* 265–273.

Williams, R. B., Poon, L. W., & Burdette, L. J. Locus of control and vasomotor response to sensory processing. *Psychosomatic Medicine,* 1977, *39,* 127–133.

Williams, R. B., Richardson, J. S., & Eichelman, B. S. Location of central nervous system neurones mediating blood pressure response of rats to shock-induced fighting. *Journal of Behavioral Medicine,* 1978, *1,* 1977–185.

Zanchetti, A. Hypothalamic control of circulation. In S. Julius & M. D. Esler (Eds.), *The nervous system in arterial hypertension.* Springfield, Ill.: Thomas, 1976.

4

Conditioning and Learning of Cardiovascular Functions

Advances in behavioral theory and experimentation in recent years suggest the need for alternative and more specific behavioral concepts allied more directly to empirical research in cardiovascular physiology (Brady, 1979; Obrist, Black, Brener, & DiCara, 1974). A comprehensive summary and overview of behavioral strategies has been presented by Cohen and Obrist (1975) in their integration of experimental findings on interactions between behavior and the cardiovascular system. They make the distinction between paradigms in which the stimuli reflexively evoke cardiovascular responses and those in which the stimuli are initially neutral but *acquire* the capacity to elicit such responses as a function of behavioral training. The first category includes the cardiovascular effects of nociceptive and noxious stimulation, exercise, and postural change. This category also includes the study of various stressful stimuli, including symbolic material, and such "integrated behavioral patterns" as feeding and sexual activity. The two integrated patterns, the defense reaction and the pattern characterized by motivated sensory intake behavior, both with relatively well-defined behavioral and cardiovascular components, are a further means of distinguishing response patterns elicited by tasks differing in their requirements, as discussed in Chapter 3.

The second category refers broadly to the study of learned or acquired change in cardiovascular functions as a consequence of particular events in the environment, such as temporal associations of environmental stimuli. The methods of classical (Pavlovian) conditioning and instrumental (operant, trial and error) conditioning constitute the most systematic and productive means of generating information about learning in the cardiovascular system. Research on cardiovascular learning has been extensive, and the purpose of this chapter is to describe how classical and operant conditioning procedures have been used to demonstrate the effects of particular environmental stimuli on cardiovascular adjustments. That is, environmental stimuli and their relationships with ongo-ing cardiovascular changes may result in altered cardiovascular responses. Such research may therefore tell us about environmental stimuli and functions as-sociated with cardiovascular disorders and may provide the basis for behavioral interventions designed to modify or normalize abnormal cardiovascular re-sponses.

In this chapter, we describe how operant and classical conditioning pro-cedures have been used in research on learning in the cardiovascular system. In both procedures, the end result is a change in the behavior of a car-diovascular response (e.g., increase in blood pressure, increase in heart rate) as a function of experience. That is, after conditioning, the cardiovascular adjustment that occurs is different from the adjustment that occurs prior to conditioning. Thus, a stimulus or situation that previously did not affect heart rate or blood pressure now results in a distinct and specific heart rate or blood pressure change, or the frequency of occurrence of such changes now varies predictably over a period of time.

Figure 4.1 shows a schematic diagram illustrating the difference between classical and operant conditioning procedures. As is suggested by the diagram, in classical conditioning, the response elicited by the unconditioned stimulus is presumed to be the same response that is learned, now elicited by the previously neutral conditioned (or conditional) stimulus. In operant condition-ing, the reinforcing stimulus can be used selectively to control any immediately preceding response. In classical conditioning, the response to be conditioned is not specifically controlled by the pairing of conditioned and unconditioned stimuli; the stimulus substitution model does not hold in a simple fashion. For example, in human classical conditioning involving the pairing of a neutral stimulus (conditioned) with an aversive stimulus (unconditioned)such as elec-tric shock, the typical heart rate conditioned response is an acceleration in rate followed by a deceleration prior to the time at which the aversive stimulus is to occur (see Brady, 1979). Other processes, such as orienting responses to the conditioned stimulus (Sokolow, 1963), concurrent respiratory and muscular changes, and other vascular and biochemical changes have a determining influ-ence in the resultant classically conditioned response. Classically conditioned changes in circulation would seem to depend on the particular requirements of the unconditioned stimulus, concomitant adjustments in somatomotor and other response components, and the balance of sympathetic and parasympathe-tic influences involved during the course of learning (see Obrist, 1981). Brady (1979) summarizes several other phenomena of particular significance for cardiovascular classical conditioning. First is the observation that single-trial classical conditioning can occur. Second, partial reinforcement (omitting the unconditioned stimulus on a selected number of trials) results in in-creasing resistance to extinction (no further presentations of the reinforcing

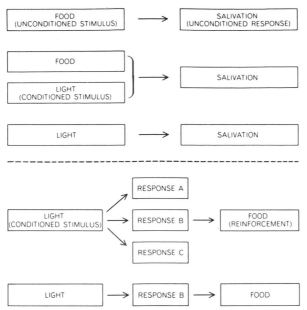

FIGURE 4.1. Top panel illustrates procedure of classical conditioning. The external stimulus (light) is paired with the unconditioned stimulus (food), resulting in the former eliciting the unconditioned response (salivation). Bottom panel illustrates procedure of operant conditioning. The reinforcement (food) can selectively control the occurrence of a specific response after several reinforcements. [From L. V. DiCara. Learning in the autonomic nervous system. *Scientific American*, 1970, 222, 36.]

stimulus). Third, discriminative learning can readily be demonstrated. That is, if two conditioned stimuli are presented, one followed consistently by the unconditioned stimulus and the other not, the magnitude of the conditioned response will be significantly greater to the former than the latter.

Although there has been considerable research on heart rate changes observed during classical conditioning in human subjects, there are only a few reports of blood pressure changes during classical conditioning in humans (De-Leon, 1972). Whitehead, Lurie, and Blackwell (1976) reported that small decreases in human systolic blood pressure could be classically conditioned in normal and hypertensive subjects. In this case, subjects were anticipating being tilted head down 15°. This conditioned stimulus elicits a decrease in blood pressure through the carotid sinus reflex. With the continuing developments of noninvasive techniques for continuous blood pressure measurement, further progress can be made in understanding conditioned effects on blood pressure as well as behavioral influences on cardiovascular reflexes and cardiovascular responses to stress.

Russian researchers have been able to produce hypertension in animals experimentally (Simonson & Brozek, 1959). A condition called *experimental neurosis* was induced by simultaneously presenting conflicting excitatory and inhibitory stimuli. The experimental neurosis was accompanied by the onset of hypertension, but this ceased when the conflict-producing situation changed. After inducing experimental neurosis in cats, Shapiro and Horn (1955) were unable to obtain signs of hypertension in these animals, although the stimulus conditions may not have been sufficiently stressful (Gutmann & Benson, 1971). In a study by Dykman and Gantt (1960), however, a conditioned hypertensive response in dogs was found to persist for over a year.

In animal research, a variation of an operant conditioning procedure involves research on cardiovascular changes associated with the performance of somatomotor responses under particular reinforcement schedules (Herd, Kelleher, Morse, & Grose, 1974). Both acute and chronic increases in blood pressure and changes in blood pressure variability can be established in these situations, which require monkeys to make continuous behavioral adjustments in the face of aversive stimuli. The research also shows that abnormal elevations in blood pressure can result and persist even after the required motor responses are no longer required. In effect, such preparatory cardiovascular responses are classically conditioned to the stimuli associated with the task and provide a behavioral source of hypertension.

A series of studies by Lown and co-workers (see Lown, de Silva, Reich, & Murawski, 1980, for a review) have elegantly demonstrated how classical conditioning may play a role in the development of a variety of cardiac arrythmias associated with sudden death. Dogs were immobilized in a sling and exposed to a repeated mild but unescapable electric shock. After 3 days of this conditioning, the dogs were exposed to the sling (conditioned stimulus) without any further electric shock. Conditional cardiac instability was observed in dogs that were recovering from induced acute myocardial infarctions when they were exposed to the sling. Using the same paradigm, dogs with normal hearts where shown to have a lower threshold for the electricity–induced repetitive extra systoles when exposed to the conditioned stimulus of the sling.

The literature in classical conditioning of cardiovascular responses is extensive, and we have cited some representative findings. However, as DiCara (1970) pointed out, the possibilities of learning (and relearning) are limited in classical conditioning because the stimulus and response must have a natural relationship to begin with. Furthermore, as we have already noted in Chapter 1, operant conditioning approaches to cardiovascular functioning allow much greater flexibility clinically in that specific cardiovascular responses can be targeted for shaping and selective conditioning. In classical conditioning, aversive stimuli are typically employed as unconditioned reinforcers. In operant conditioning, both positive and negative stimuli are utilized to reinforce the appropriate response. From the standpoint of treatment and rehabilitation, operant conditioning and biofeedback techniques appear to have a much greater potential than classical conditioning techniques. For these reasons, we have devoted the bulk of this chapter to biofeedback and operant conditioning of cardiovascular responses.

BIOFEEDBACK AND OPERANT CONDITIONING
OF CARDIOVASCULAR FUNCTIONS

The first important discussion of the concept of biofeedback was in Razran's monograph (1961) on research in the Soviet Union and Eastern Europe concerned with interoceptive conditioning, semantic conditioning, and the orienting reflex. Razran described an experiment by Lisina indicating that subjects could learn to control their vasomotor activity to avoid noxious stimulation, but only under the condition of observing their own polygraph record of the continuous physiological changes. The procedure of observing a visual, auditory, tactile, or other sensory representation of one's own physiological responses, locked in time to the actual occurrence of these responses, is the essence of the biofeedback method. The goal of biofeedback is to enable the individual to gain voluntary control over such responses, to increase or decrease response levels, rate of occurrence, or other characteristics. It is not simply the presentation of biofeedback as information that leads to such control, but rather that the information is utilized by the individual in some manner to modify his or her behavior so as to achieve such control. The biofeedback serves to reinforce the desired physiological changes.

Aside from the early Soviet research on vascular activity, a number of other investigations showed that minute muscle twitches and other isolated activities of single motor units could be voluntarily controlled by means of biofeedback and associated reinforcement for the appropriate changes. In these cases, electromyographic (EMG) recordings of muscle activities were used to produce visual or auditory displays of physiological responses (Basmajian, 1963; Hefferline, Keenan, & Harford, 1959). With regard to central nervous system (CNS) responses, the early investigations of Kamiya (1969) on the control of alpha electroencephalogram (EEG) activity (8–12 Hz) stimulated much research to follow. Kamiya was concerned with the ability of subjects to discriminate such changes, and then went on to study the ability of subjects to increase or decrease this activity. Other laboratories reported that the human electrodermal response, either measured as a skin resistance or skin potential change, could be relatively increased or decreased in frequency by contingent reinforcement (Fowler & Kimmel, 1962; Johnson, 1963; D. Shapiro, Crider, & Tursky, 1964).

One study in this series (D. Shapiro *et al.*, 1964) is emphasized because it illustrates the methodology of biofeedback research. A spontaneous fluctuation of palmar skin potential of a given amplitude was selected as the response to be brought under control. All subjects were told that the purpose of the experiment was to study the effectiveness of various devices for measuring thought processes. They were instructed that each time the apparatus detected an "emotional thought" they would hear a tone and earn some money. One group of subjects was given a reward each time a skin potential response occurred; a second group was given the same number of rewards but at times when the response was absent. The first group showed increases in response rate relative to the second group, which showed a response decrement. The fact that the same reward, with instructions held constant, could be used either to enhance *or* to diminish the autonomic response eliminated the explanation that the eliciting effect of the reinforcer could account for the observed differences. Learned variations in electrodermal response rate were found not to be associated with such physiologically related functions as skin potential level and heart rate. Nor were the variations associated with changes in respiration. Response contingent and nonresponse contingent subjects reported the same moderate relationship between the reinforcer (tone indicating bonus) and their thoughts or ideation; level of involvement in the task was also about the same for the two groups.

The basic implication of the study was that the feedback and associated reinforcement were critical in selecting out a given response and shaping its frequency, while at the same time presumably related responses did not covary. If an operant procedure could have a selective effect on an autonomically mediated behavior, it made a convincing argument for the value of exploring autonomic regulation of specific functions or patterns of functions with these methods. Moreover, if a given response is reinforced, the degree to which other presumably related responses change in the same direction could indicate their functional relationship.

Although the foundations for biofeedback research were laid down in these early human investigations, the animal research of Miller, DiCara, and associates (Miller, 1969) was a major influence in subsequent research. Their goal was to establish that operant conditioning of heart rate and other visceral functions was not necessarily dependent on somatomotor activity. They used curare to paralyze animals, examined the degree to which the animals could learn to control visceral activities with operant conditioning, and employed brain stimulation or shock escape and avoidance as reinforcers. Their initial results were positive in many experiments in rats and cats. Rather substantial increases and decreases in physiological response rate were obtained in the curarized animals (Miller, 1969). However, difficulties in replicating these experiments resulted in a slowing down of animal research (Miller & Dworkin, 1974; Roberts, 1978). The use of muscular paralysis does not rule out the influence of CNS motor centers on visceral activities (Black, 1972; Obrist, 1976; Obrist, Howard, Lawler, Galosy, Meyers, & Gaebelein, 1974). Researchers concluded that there can be some independence of somatic and autonomic activities and that peripheral muscular activity can probably be ruled out as a *necessary* requirement for learned visceral control. On the other hand, somatomotor and autonomic functions often vary together according to different behavioral settings and demands (Cohen & Obrist, 1975; Obrist, 1976). They are coupled together in various ways at all levels of the nervous system. Alternative approaches in animal research are to assess physiological mechanisms by the use of lesions and ablations, biochemical and drug influences, and so on. Studies of humans with neurological and neuromuscular diseases are also pertinent (Miller, 1975; Pickering, Brucker, Frankel, Mathias, Dworkin, & Miller, 1977). From a purely clinical standpoint, the fact that self-regulation is mediated by somatomotor or cognitive processes is of no consequence so long as the desired goal of physiological change can be achieved and maintained and there are no unwanted side effects of such mediating processes. Moreover, the mediational activities can be used positively to facilitate the development of physiological control.

The single most remarkable feature of biofeedback is its potential for selective control of specific responses or patterns of response, and this feature may be of particular significance in the management of cardiovascular disorders (see following sections). Alternative methods of behavioral control (e.g., simple relaxation, specific suggestions) can possibly be used to achieve comparable specificity, although the biofeedback approach appears to offer the most direct and efficient way to achieve control over patterns of physiological responses. Research on the control of patterns of visceral and somatomotor activity would also serve to elucidate the biologic and behavioral significance of the defense reaction, sensory processing reaction, or other integrated biologic response patterns (see Chapter 3).

The following sections will review selective research on cardiovascular functions that provides an empirical foundation for the application of biofeedback (and related behavioral approaches) in the treatment of cardiovascular disorders.

Blood Pressure

Basic research on biofeedback in the regulation of blood pressure includes data from animal and human experiments. In the curarized rat, instrumental conditioning of systolic blood pressure was demonstrated using shock escape and avoidance (DiCara & Miller, 1968b). Learned changes in pressure were about 20% of baseline in both increase and decrease directions, and they were not associated with changes in heart rate or rectal temperature. In a subsequent study in noncurarized rats, changes obtained were about 5% of baseline (Pappas, DiCara, & Miller, 1970). Diastolic pressure elevations of large magnitude (50–60 mm Hg) were obtained in the rhesus monkey using shock avoidance response (Plumlee, 1969). In the baboon, substantial elevations in blood pressure were established by an operant procedure in which food delivery and shock avoidance were made contingent upon increases in diastolic pressure (Harris, Findley, & Brady, 1971; Harris, Gilliam, Findley, & Brady, 1973). In their more recent work, Harris and co-workers reported sustained increases of about 30–40 mm Hg in both systolic and diastolic blood pressure. The changes in blood pressure were associated with elevated but progressively decreasing heart rates (Harris & Brady, 1974). Long-term studies of such cardiovascular control in primates and associated physiological mechanisms are discussed further in Harris and Brady (1977).

Most of the human studies on blood pressure control with biofeedback methods follow the procedures first described in D. Shapiro, Tursky, Gershon, and Stern (1969). The constant-cuff technique was devised to obtain a relative measure of blood pressure on each beat of the heart in order to provide continuous feedback to subjects. Initial studies with the constant-cuff method attempted to determine whether normal volunteer subjects could learn to modify their systolic or diastolic blood pressure. In these studies, subjects were told that the feedback represented information about a physiological response usually considered involuntary. Subjects were told to make the feedback stimulus occur as much as possible and thereby to earn as many rewards as possible. They were not told that the feedback was being given for changes in blood pressure, nor were they told whether to increase it or decrease it. This procedure controlled for any results that are due to the natural ability of subjects to control their pressure "voluntarily," and tested the specific effects of feedback and reward contingency. Voluntary control of blood pressure and other circulatory changes has been reported in some individuals (Ogden & Shock, 1939). Such voluntary control of blood pressure unassisted by external feedback could not be demonstrated in a sample of normal subjects (Brener, 1974; D. Shapiro, 1973).

To summarize the results, normal subjects were able to modify their blood pressure with feedback and reward. Average differences in systolic pressure between increase and decrease conditions for groups of subjects at the end of a single session of training varied from 3 to 10% of baseline (D. Shapiro *et al.,* 1969). The best results were obtained for diastolic pressure (D. Shapiro,

Schwartz, & Tursky, 1972), with individuals showing increases of up to 25% and decreases of up to 15% of baseline values. Heart rate was not associated with learned changes in systolic pressure, and systolic pressure was not associated with learned changes in heart rate (D. Shapiro, Tursky, & Schwartz, 1970b). However, Fey and Lindholm (1975) reported that heart rate increased or decreased in groups receiving contingent feedback for increasing and for decreasing systolic blood pressure, respectively. Brener (1974), citing data in which continuous recordings of heart rate, chin EMG, and respiratory activity were obtained while subjects were given both increase and decrease feedback training for diastolic blood pressure, reported that training effects were specific to blood pressure. However, D. Shapiro *et al.,* (1972) reported that heart rate was not independent of learned changes in diastolic pressure. Further evidence is needed on the specificity of control, particularly on associated changes that occur in the conditioning process. Information is critical about such side effects if these techniques are to be employed effectively in the behavioral management of blood pressure.

Schwartz (1972) hypothesized that, when feedback is given for one response, simultaneous learning of other responses will depend on the degree to which these other responses are directly associated with the response for which feedback is given. He developed an on-line procedure for tracking both phasic and tonic patterns of blood pressure and heart rate in real time and showed that subjects could learn to control patterns of simultaneous changes in both functions. Subjects learned to integrate systolic blood pressure and heart rate (i.e., make both increase or both decrease simultaneously) and to some extent to differentiate both functions (i.e., make one increase and the other decrease simultaneously). Further analysis of the patterning of both functions over time, of natural tonic reactivity in this situation, and of homeostatic mechanisms made it possible to predict the extent and time course of pattern learning in the different conditions (Schwartz, 1974). Subjective reports of a "relaxed" state were associated with learned reductions in both systolic pressure and heart rate.

Although the average curves suggest that it is easier to obtain reductions rather than increases in pressure in a single session (D. Shapiro *et al.,* 1969), further data under conditions of random reinforcement indicated a tendency for baseline pressure values to habituate over time (D. Shapiro, Tursky, & Schwartz, 1970a). Unpublished data (D. Shapiro, Note 1) indicated that the same pattern of pressure reduction occurs whether subjects try to reduce their pressure with or without feedback or simply rest in the laboratory and do nothing. On the other hand, Fey and Lindholm (1975), using the constant-cuff method and unrestricted subjects, reported reliable decreases in systolic blood pressure as compared with no changes in no-feedback, random, or increase training groups. Surwit, Hager, and Feldman (1977) conducted a study in which normal subjects were instructed to increase and decrease their blood pressure. Subjects were given either contingent beat-to-beat feedback, noncontingent beat-to-beat feedback, noncontingent feedback randomly associated with the heartbeat, or no feedback at all. No clear differences between training conditions were observed in this one-session study. This calls into question the utility of feedback when instructions are given. Blood pressure increases were easier to obtain than blood pressure decreases.

As in the case of heart rate, the processes involved in increasing blood pressure may be different from those involved in decreasing pressure (Engel, 1972; Lang & Twentyman, 1974). In normal subjects, typical resting pressures are close to minimal waking values, but there is a potential for large increases above baseline. For individuals having significantly elevated pressure levels, significant decreases may be more likely.

All told, blood pressure biofeedback research suggests that blood pressure can be self-regulated by normal subjects with a fair degree of consistency and specificity. The degree of change achieved, especially in a decrease direction, is relatively small. Most of the human research consists of one-session experiments in subjects already low in pressure to begin with. More work is needed to determine whether larger and persistent changes can be brought about with long-term training. Pattern feedback techniques need to be exploited, particularly with the aid of computer techniques. The effects on blood pressure of biofeedback for other cardiovascular parameters (e.g. heart rate, skin blood flow, muscle blood flow) also needs to be explored more systematically.

Other, more refined techniques of measuring blood pressure on a continuous basis may also serve to advance research on the control of blood pressure. We developed a system for the automatic tracking of blood pressure, which provides a more precise estimate of systolic (or diastolic) blood pressure at each successive heartbeat (D. Shapiro, Greenstadt, Lane, & Rubinstein, 1981). For systolic pressure, the system has been validated against simultaneous intraarterial pressure recording (D. Shapiro et al., 1981) and has been used effectively in several biofeedback studies (Holroyd, Nuechterlein, Shapiro, & Ward, 1979; D. Shapiro, Reeves, Greenstadt, Dolan, Cobb, & Lane, 1979). Along with other noninvasive cardiovascular measurement techniques (see Chapter 2), the ability to monitor blood pressure on a continuous basis can help advance research on cardiovascular–behavioral interactions.

Pulse Wave Velocity

The previously mentioned studies have attempted to modify blood pressure, mainly using variations of the constant-cuff pressure technique (D. Shapiro *et al.,* 1969). However, the cuff method requires periodic and/or sustained limb occlusions, and such occlusions may result in discomfort to subjects. Moreover, the cuff has to be deflated about every minute, resulting in discontinuous recordings. Advances in the measurement of pulse wave velocity suggest an alternative to cuff methods. Pulse wave velocity is the rate of propagation of a pressure pulse through the arteries; it also relates to the size of the arteries and their distensibility. It can be evaluated by timing the interval between the arrival of a pulse at two different points along the same artery (Gribbin, Steptoe, & Sleight, 1976) or by measuring the time between the R-wave of the electrocardiogram (EKG) and the arrival of the pulse at the brachial or radial artery (Williams & Williams, 1965). Investigators employ a measure of velocity (distance per time) or pulse transit time (PTT) itself. Substantial correlations have been reported between PTT and mean arterial pressure as measured by arterial cannulation (Steptoe, Smulyan, & Gribbin, 1976) or systolic pressure as measured by a standard cuff method (Obrist, Langer, & Grignolo, 1977). Steptoe and Johnston (1976) demonstrated that voluntary control of PTT is possible to some degree with instructions only and to a larger degree with PTT feedback. They reported reliable differences in PTT, assumed to be equivalent to over 11 mm Hg in blood pressure, between increase and decrease PTT feedback conditions. Changes in PTT did not seem to be systematically related to changes in heart rate.

The precise nature of the relationship between PTT and blood pressure—whether systolic, diastolic, or mean—is uncertain at this time. The correlations reported between PTT and blood pressure may derive from their common association with other processes. Thus, the R-wave to peripheral pulse time is composed of the preejection period of the cardiac cycle as well as the time for propagation of the pulse through the arteries. A study by Obrist and co-workers (Obrist, Light, McCubbin, Hutcheson, & Hoffer, 1979) concluded that PTT was greatly influenced by myocardial sympathetic excitation and to a lesser degree by vascular processes. Although PTT (measured from R-wave to a peripheral pulse) may not uniquely index blood pressure, it is nonetheless a practical noninvasive measure of cardiovascular function and merits further attention.

Heart Rate

There is a large literature on the use of biofeedback in the voluntary regulation of heart rate. Heart rate changes have been repeatedly demonstrated in animals (DiCara & Miller, 1968a; Miller & DiCara, 1967; Trowill, 1967) and in humans (Brener & Hothersall, 1966; Engel & Hansen, 1966; Hnatiow & Lang, 1965; D. Shapiro *et al.,* 1970b). Although procedures for blood pressure feedback are extremely complicated, heart rate is an easy function to monitor.

With the use of surface electrodes, heart rate can be monitored continuously and presented either as an analog function of rate or heart period (i.e., the time between R-waves in the EKG) or as a dichotomous binary signal indicating whether or not the subject is above or below criterion on each beat of the heart.

Studies have reported average heart rate increases in excess of 10 beats per minute (bpm) (Blanchard, Young, Scott, & Haynes, 1974; Colgan, 1977; Obrist, Galosy, Lawler, Gaebelein, Howard, & Shanks, 1975). Wells (1973) reported that six out of nine subjects produced heart rate increases of greater than 15 bpm. The remainder of this sample failed to produce heart rate increases above 7 bpm. This dichotomy of ability is characteristic of the great individual differences reported by most investigators exploring heart rate control (Bell & Schwartz, 1975; Colgan, 1977; Stephens, Harris, Brady, & Shaffer, 1975).

Although individual differences appear to play a role in voluntary heart rate slowing, subjects seem less able to decrease their heart rate from a stable baseline than to increase their heart rate. Only a few studies (Colgan, 1977; Sirota, Schwartz, & Shapiro, 1974, 1976) have reported mean heart rate decreases of greater than 5 bpm. However, the data from the Sirota *et al.* studies are complicated by the fact that only 5-min adaptation periods are used, and subjects are exposed to the threat of a noxious stimulus during the course of training. The discrepancy between the ability of subjects to increase and decrease their heart rate voluntarily when provided with heart rate feedback has led to speculations that heart rate increases and decreases might be mediated by different physiological mechanisms (Bell & Schwartz, 1975; Lang, Troyer, Twentyman, & Gatchel, 1975).

As with blood pressure, investigators have asked the question as to whether or not heart rate can be manipulated with equal facility both with and without feedback in instructed subjects. Bergman and Johnson (1971) demonstrated that heart rate could be voluntarily controlled to some degree without feedback. Furthermore, Bergman and Johnson (1972) reported that the addition of heart rate feedback did not significantly improve the performance of subjects simply instructed to control their heart rate. More recently, studies have reported that increases in heart rate are significantly larger in subjects given feedback as well as instructional control (Bell & Schwartz, 1975; Davidson & Schwartz, 1976; Lang & Twentyman, 1974, 1976). In the control of heart rate decreases, the facilitatory effect of feedback is not as clear (Davidson & Schwartz, 1976; Young & Blanchard, 1974).

Heart rate feedback is presented either as an analog or binary signal. Analog signals usually consist of some type of visual display in which the change of the signal is proportional to the heart rate change. Binary signals provide the subject with yes–no information on a beat-by-beat or time-period basis. This type of feedback is computed by setting a criterion of rate or interbeat interval and then comparing the ongoing heart rate to this criterion during discrete time periods. The subject then sees a signal informing him whether or not he is higher or lower than this target at any given point in time. Three of five studies comparing analog to binary feedback have demonstrated a clear superiority for analog feedback in increasing heart rate (Blanchard *et al.,* 1974; Colgan, 1977; Lang & Twentyman, 1974; Manuck, Levenson, Hinrichsen, & Gryll, 1975; Young & Blanchard, 1974).

Peripheral Vasomotor Activity

Control of digital skin temperature through biofeedback and instrumental learning has been cited as a clinical tool for the control of migraine headaches (Sargent, Green, & Walters, 1973) and Raynaud's disease (Surwit, 1973) (see Chapters 7 and 8). Since the peripheral vasculature is innervated exclusively by the sympathetic nervous system (Patton, 1965), control of digital temperature provides one of the clearest examples of voluntary control of the sympathetic nervous system available in human experimentation. Indeed, the earliest demonstration that an autonomic response may be learned with the aid of feedback occurred in the vasomotor system (Lisina, 1958/1965).

This investigation was attempting to train subjects to vasodilate in the forearm in order to escape an electric shock. Lisina observed that subjects were unable to learn the response until they were allowed to watch the strip chart recording of the plethysmograph to which they were connected. Using this form of feedback, subjects readily learned to vasoconstrict in order to escape shock. Although Katkin and Murray (1968) noted that Lisina's demonstration of forearm blood flow control could be dismissed as a function of respiratory maneuvers, Synder and Noble (1968) conducted an experiment that circumvented this criticism. Using the digital plethysmograph they demonstrated that subjects could learn to voluntarily vasoconstrict in the digits of the hands while skeletal muscle activity was controlled. Most of the research concerning voluntary control of peripheral vasomotor responses utilizes skin temperature as the dependent variable. The relationship of skin temperature to blood flow is nonlinear. Temperature rises with blood flow until it approaches core temperature (36–37°C). At that point, blood flow can increase markedly while skin temperature will not change. Therefore, there are distinct limitations to this variable. However, because skin temperature is easily measurable, as well as quantifiable, it has been used in the majority of studies investigating voluntary control of digital blood flow. As long as one keeps in mind the ceiling effect that confounds this measure, the results of studies utilizing skin temperature as a measure of blood flow are usually interpretable.

Hadfield (1920) reported control of skin temperature using eidetic imagery. Subjects were told to imagine that their hands were warm or cold and corresponding temperature changes were observed. Maslach, Marshall, and Zimbardo (1972) demonstrated that subjects could learn to control digital skin temperature through the use of hypnosis. All hypnotized subjects demonstrated an ability to produce bilateral changes in digital skin temperature. Temperature decreases were easier to produce and were generally larger than temperature increases. While the largest decrease in temperature from baseline under hypnosis was 7°C, the largest increase observed was only 2°C. Subjects who were not hypnotized were unable to show significant changes in temperature. A. Roberts, Kewman, and MacDonald (1973) trained subjects to control skin temperature differentially in the digits of two hands with the aid of hypnosis and feedback. In 1975, A. Roberts, Schuler, Bacon, Zimmerman, and Patterson demonstrated that neither hypnotic susceptibility nor hypnosis were necessary for this effect to occur if differential feedback of the temperature between two hands was provided. Steptoe, Mathews, and Johnston (1974) were able to train human subjects to produce small but reliable (.3°C) differences in temperature between the two earlobes. A surgical collar fitted to each subject prevented movement of the head toward the trunk. However, measures of EMG activity from the mastoid area revealed a differential effect of EMG that approached significance. The muscular activity seemed to increase in the side of the head that the subjects were trying to warm.

Keefe (1975) used visual and auditory feedback to train subjects to differentially increase finger temperature from forehead skin temperature. Four subjects were instructed to raise the temperature of the digit, while another group of four subjects was instructed to lower the temperature of the digit in relation to the forehead. After 12 sessions of training, statistically significant bidirectional changes in differential temperature were obtained. Subjects in the increase group showed an average increase in differential skin temperature of up to 1.9°F over the 10-min feedback period. Subjects in the decrease group showed a decrease in temperature of up to 1.5°F. Absolute skin temperature varied with differential temperature. Surwit, Shapiro, and Feld (1976) trained 16 subjects to either increase or decrease absolute digital skin temperature. Subjects were given 2 baseline sessions and up to 9 training sessions. Feedback was presented from analog panel meters and subjects were reinforced with 25 cents per .1°C change in the appropriate direction. No particular strategies or instructions were given to the subjects other than the response and direction in which their training was to occur. Subjects were able to show an average decrease of up to 2°C over a 25-min training period. Some subjects were able to show as much as a 10°C drop per session. In contrast to this, learning to increase skin temperature appeared to be much more difficult. Subjects reinforced for increases in skin temperature showed average increases of only .25°C, with the largest increase being 3.5°C (see Figure 4.2). Temperature changes appeared bilaterally and were not specific to the training site (nondominant hand). Data from both girth and reflectance plethysmographs indicated that pulse amplitude changed in the expected direction with temperature. Interestingly, heart rate tended to increase over days of training in subjects trained to increase skin temperature. Subjects trained to decrease skin temperature showed heart rate decline over days of training. There appeared to be no advantage in extending the training from 5 to 9 days. Because skin temperatures in the group of subjects trained to vasodilate tended to approach core temperature (i.e., they reach 34–35°C), a second experiment was designed in which the ambient temperature of the laboratory was lowered in order to lower basal digital temperature of the subjects trying to vasodilate. Eight subjects were given the same training procedure as before. However, subjects were still unable to show dramatic increases of skin temperature with feedback. Surwit *et al.*, (1976) concluded that the reason subjects had more difficulty raising skin temperature than lowering it might have to do with the feedback situation itself. Specifically, they noted that the introduction of feedback dropped digital skin temperature over 3°C from resting baseline. This vasoconstriction in response to stimulation was similar to that reported by Sokolow (1963) in his description of the orienting reflex. Surwit *et al.* (1976) also noted that the apparent differential ability to increase as opposed to decrease arousal-like behavior is consistent with results of studies on a voluntary control of blood pressure and heart rate (Blanchard & Young, 1973), salivation (Wells, *et al.*,

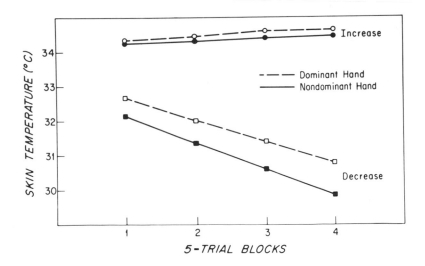

FIGURE 4.2. Mean digital temperature over trial blocks for increase and decrease groups. Each point is collapsed over 5 days of training for 8 subjects. [From R. S. Surwit, D. Shapiro, & J. L. Feld. Digital temperature autoregulation and associated cardiovascular changes. *Psychophysiology*, 1976, *13*, 242.]

1973), and occipital alpha control (Paskowitz & Orne, 1974). It was thus hypothesized that increases in sympathetic activity producing such responses as vasoconstriction are easier to learn with the biofeedback paradigm than decreases in sympathetic activity.

Lynch, Hamma, Kohn, and Miller (1976) also reported difficulty in obtaining control of peripheral skin temperature in adults. However, they were able to achieve modest success in training small changes in differential temperature between the right and the left hands using visual feedback and rewards in children. Three of the four children learned to differentially vasoconstrict and reduce the temperature of the right and the left hand. In an extension of this study, one child was trained to decrease the temperature of two adjacent digits differentially. It is of interest that in the study by Lynch *et al.* (1976) and in the studies by A. Roberts *et al.* (1973, 1975), subjects were able to produce differential changes by inducing vasoconstriction in the two sites at different rates. No investigator has succeeded in producing vasodilatation in one limb while simultaneously inducing vasoconstriction in the other. Keefe and Gardner (1979) also reported that the effects of skin temperature training seemed to peak at 5 sessions. In this experiment, subjects were given 5 or 20 sessions of feedback to either increase or decrease skin temperature. In both conditions, subjects reached an asymptomatic level of performance by session 3, with negligible increases in voluntary vasoconstriction or vasodilatation with extended training.

The most dramatic changes in skin temperature through the use of temperature feedback have been reported by Taub and Emurian (1976). In this study, 8 males and 13 females participated in a varied number of training sessions with skin temperature feedback from the web-dorsum of the subject's dominant hand. Feedback was provided by a variable-intensity light and, as in the study by Surwit *et al.* (1976), subjects were paid 25 cents for each .25°C in the appropriate direction. The authors did not specify whether this reinforcement was net change from initial baseline or simply from the previous immediate temperature. All subjects were trained for a minimum of 4 days, and some were trained for up to 6 days. Each subject received one 45-min baseline session prior to training. Although Taub often emphasizes the performance of several of his individual subjects (Taub & Emurian, 1976), the parametric data from this study are quite similar to those of Surwit *et al.* (1976). Subjects trained to decrease their temperature showed larger changes in the appropriate direction than subjects trained to increase their temperature. On the initial training day, subjects trained to decrease temperature showed a mean decrease of 2.25°F, whereas subjects trained to increase their temperature showed a mean increase of 1°F. Because Surwit *et al.* (1976) demonstrated that temperature could continue to increase over 2 baseline days and Taub only used 1 baseline day, any difference between the two studies could easily be attributed to habituation. Taub also gave his subjects autogenic phrases to aid in vasodilatation. Nevertheless, skin temperature increases were harder to obtain than skin temperature decreases.

Keefe and Gardner (1979) trained 40 male college students with the aid of skin temperature feedback and instructions. Half of the subjects were told that feedback was for digital skin temperature changes, while the remaining half were not. The subjects who had knowledge of the target response were able to produce significant within-session changes in skin temperature consistently after 6 sessions of training, whereas subjects who were uninformed as to the nature of the response were able to produce similar changes only after 11 sessions of training. As in previous work, skin temperature changes were modest ($\overline{X} = 1.5°F$) in either the increase or the decrease direction.

EFFECTS OF BIOFEEDBACK ON
COMPLEX PHYSIOLOGICAL SYSTEMS

In applying biofeedback or instrumental learning techniques, it must be remembered that one is dealing with complex physiological systems and not one simple response. This is particularly true in the case of cardiovascular responses. Often, the response one chooses to modify is the end product of many interacting processes, all of which might be measurable and trainable in and of themselves. Optimal manipulation of a system may therefore be achieved by manipulating underlying physiological processes directly rather than the gross response that constitutes the target behavior (Shapiro & Surwit, 1976). This is probably best illustrated by the case of blood pressure control.

Figure 4.3 is a schematic diagram summarizing the basic physiological processes that affect arterial blood pressure. As can be seen, mean arterial pressure is determined by cardiac output and total peripheral resistance. Though cardiac output and peripheral resistance are somewhat interrelated functions, they can also be seen to be independent in the etiology of hypertension. For instance, patients suffering from sustained hypertension are known to have increased peripheral resistance but normal cardiac output, whereas patients displaying labile hypertension show increased cardiac output and normal peripheral resistance. When biofeedback is used for treating hypertension, different procedures might be indicated depending upon the stage of hypertension. For example, since heart rate is one component of cardiac output, labile hypertensives might benefit more than fixed hypertensives from a combination of blood pressure and heart rate feedback, since high cardiac output is one

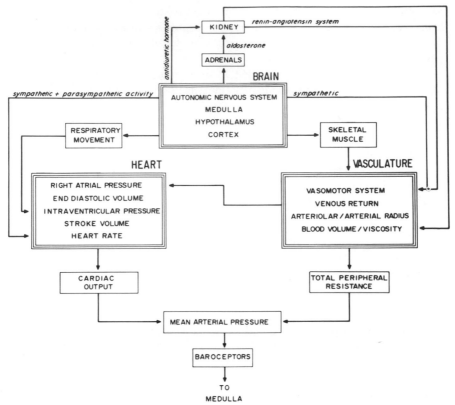

FIGURE 4.3. Schematic diagram summarizing the physiological mechanisms involved in the regulation of arterial blood pressure. The diagram oversimplifies the process involved in order to provide a general overview of mechanisms most relevant to behavioral manipulation. Boxes labeled Heart, Brain, and Vasculature each contain a subset of relevant systems and functions. While these are not necessarily temporally or functionally related in the order presented, the outside arrows indicate the site at which other systems exert their influence on the system described in the box. The reader should note the numerous and diverse pathways through which behavioral control over blood pressure could be exerted. For example, relaxation techniques acting on the muscles could have their main effect on the vasculature, producing a decrease in peripheral resistance. Yogic exercises emphasizing breath control might have their main effect on cardiac output by changing intraventricular pressure. While the diagram suggests that a feedback approach including both cardiac and vascular parameters would be most efficacious, it illustrates how verbal instruction acting on the cortex might also be seen to affect blood pressure. [From D. Shapiro & R. Surwit. Learned control of physiological function and disease. In H. Leitenberg (Ed.), *Handbook of behavior modification and behavior therapy* (Englewood Cliffs, N.J.: Prentice-Hall, 1976). © 1976 by Prentice-Hall, Inc. Reprinted by permission of Prentice-Hall, Inc., Englewood Cliffs, New Jersey.]

characteristic of their disorder. Heart rate feedback, however, would not be indicated for fixed hypertensives, since their cardiac output is normal. For them, some combination of pressure and muscle tension might be useful.

Those conducting research on the application of biofeedback to hypertension should be cognizant of the multitude of ways in which pressure can be reduced—some of which may not be particularly therapeutic. Since instrumental control of urine formation may be possible (Miller & DiCara, 1967), one might want to check that patients were not decreasing their blood pressure by reducing their urine volume. Such laboratory induced changes would be transient, lasting only until the patient had a drink of water. It is also possible that patients could learn to control cardiac output through manipulation of respiration and intrathoracic pressure. Again, such changes are unlikely to be generalized to outside the laboratory. Longer lasting changes might be achieved through training aspects of peripheral resistance or cardiac output.

Research suggests that the most useful method of control of blood pressure might be decrease of sympathetic activity. It may be hypothesized that *general* physiological functions such as sympathetic activity are more readily subject to control because they involve a number of common nervous pathways that are integrated at higher levels of the nervous system. Thus, Schwartz (1972) found larger decreases (or increases) in heart rate *and* systolic blood pressure when feedback and rewards were given for the simultaneous occurrence of decreases (or increases) in *both,* as compared to earlier results when only one or the other function was reinforced (D. Shapiro *et al.,* 1970b).

On the other hand, modifying a global pattern of activity means that some unwanted accompanying change may be augmented. While further analysis of data from an earlier study (Shapiro *et al.,* 1972) suggest that it is difficult to dissociate such closely integrated responses as diastolic pressure and heart rate with a small amount of training, such response discrimination is theoretically possible unless there are rigid constraints of anatomy or physiology. The strategy of training would be to go from the general to the specific, at first utilizing as many common response tendencies and then selectively controlling the specific response independently of the others.

CONCLUSIONS

Classical and operant conditioning methods have served to generate a vast literature on the degree to which cardiovascular responses can be modified by experience, that is, the degree to which cardiovascular responses can be learned. The evidence is clear that behavior and experience exert a significant influence on the cardiovascular system, not only in terms of transient or short-term responses to stimuli, but also in terms of relatively permanent alterations of cardiovascular response levels. Thus, conditioning methods have been utilized to determine whether abnormal response levels can be produced by behavioral and environmental manipulation. This provokes a critical test of the idea that the environment can produce cardiovascular disorders and a means of investigating in animal studies the course of such disorders and associated hemodynamic and biochemical changes. Conditioning methods can also be utilized to investigate disease processes in animals with CNS lesions or other organ derangements, that is, to investigate certain behavioral–biologic interactions. Further examples of animal behavioral models of cardiovascular disease are discussed in Chapter 6. Finally, the research methods and findings presented in this chapter provide a major source of fundamental knowledge relevant to the prevention and treatment of cardiovascular disorders by means of behavioral approaches.

REFERENCE NOTE

1. Shapiro, D. Unpublished data, 1972.

REFERENCES

Basmajian, J. V. Control and training of individual motor units. *Science,* 1963, *141,* 440–441.
Bell, I. R., & Schwartz, G. E. Voluntary control and reactivity of human heart rate. *Psychophysiology,* 1975, *12,* 339–348.
Bergman, J. S., & Johnson, H. J. The effects of instructional set and autonomic perception on cardiac control. *Psychophysiology,* 1971, *8,* 180–190.
Bergman, J. S., & Johnson, H. J. Sources of information which affect training and raising of heart rate. *Psychophysiology,* 1972, *9,* 30–39.
Black, A. H. The operant conditioning of central nervous system electrical activity. In G. H. Bower (Ed.), *The psychology of learning and motivation: Advances in research and theory.* New York: Academic Press, 1972.
Blanchard, E. B., & Young, L. D. Self-control of cardiac functioning: A promise as yet unfulfilled. *Psychology Bulletin,* 1973, *79* 145–163.
Blanchard, E. B., Young, L. D., Scott, R. W., & Haynes, M. R. Differential effects of feedback and reinforcement in voluntary acceleration of human heart rate. *Perceptual and Motor Skills,* 1974, *38,* 683–691.
Brady, J. B. Learning and conditioning. In O. F. Pomerleau & J. P. Brady (Eds.), *Behavioral medicine: Theory and practice.* Baltimore: Williams & Wilkins, 1979.
Brener, J. A general model of voluntary control applied to the phenomena of learned cardiovascular change. In P. A. Obrist, A. H. Black, J. Brener, & L. V. DiCara (Eds.), *Cardiovascular psychophysiology.* Chicago: Aldine, 1974.

Brener, J., & Hothersall, D. Heart rate control under conditions of augmented sensory feedback. *Psychophysiology*, 1966, *3*, 23–28.

Cohen, D. H., & Obrist, P. A. Interactions between behavior and the cardiovascular system. *Circulation Research*, 1975, *37*, 693–706.

Colgan, M. Effects of binary and proportional feedback on bidirectional control of heart rate. *Psychophysiology*, 1977, *14*, 187–191.

Davidson, R. J., & Schwartz, G. E. The psychobiology of relaxation and related states: A multi-process theory. In D. I. Mostofsky (Ed.), *Behavior control and modification of physiological activity*. Englewood Cliffs, N.J.: Prentice-Hall, 1976.

DeLeon, G. Classical conditioning and extinction of human systolic blood pressure. *Conditioned Reflex*, 1972, *7*, 193–209.

DiCara, L. V. Learning in the autonomic nervous system. *Scientific American*, 1970, *222*, 30–39.

DiCara, L. V., & Miller, N. E. Changes in heart rate instrumentally learned by curarized rats as avoidance responses. *Journal of Comparative and Physiological Psychology*, 1968, *65*, 8–12. (a)

DiCara, L. V., & Miller, N. E. Instrumental learning of systolic blood pressure responses by curarized rats: Dissociation of cardiac and vascular changes. *Psychosomatic Medicine*, 1968, *30*, 489–494. (b)

Dykman, R. A., & Gantt, W. H. Experimental psychogenic hypertension: Blood pressure changes conditioned to painful stimuli (Schizokinesis). *Bulletin of Johns Hopkins Hospital*, 1960, *107*, 72–89.

Engel, B. T. Operant conditioning of cardiac function: A status report. *Psychophysiology*, 1972, *9*, 161–177.

Engel, B. T., & Hansen, S. P. Operant conditioning of heart rate slowing. *Psychophysiology*, 1966, *3*, 176–187.

Fey, S. G., & Lindholm, E. Systolic blood pressure and heart rate changes during three sessions involving biofeedback or no feedback. *Psychophysiology*, 1975, *12*, 513–519.

Fowler, R. L., & Kimmel, H. D. Operant conditioning of the GSR. *Journal of Experimental Psychology*, 1962, *63*, 563–567.

Gribbin, B., Steptoe, A., & Sleight, P. Pulse wave velocity as a measure of blood pressure change. *Psychophysiology*, 1976, *13*, 86–90.

Gutmann, M. C., & Benson, H. Interaction of environmental factors and systemic arterial blood pressure: A review. *Medicine*, 1971, *50*, 543–553.

Hadfield, A. The influence of suggestion on body temperature, *Lancet*, 1920, *2*, 82–89.

Harris, A. H., & Brady, J. B. Animal learning—Visceral and autonomic conditioning. In M. R. Rosenzweig & L. W. Porter (Eds.), *Annual review of psychology* (Vol. 25). Palo Alto: Annual Reviews, 1974.

Harris, A. H., & Brady, J. B. Long-term studies of cardiovascular control in primates. In G. E. Schwartz & J. Beatty (Eds.), *Biofeedback: Theory and research*. New York: Academic Press, 1977.

Harris, A. H., Findley, J. D., & Brady, J. B. Instrumental conditioning of blood pressure elevations in the baboon. *Conditioned Reflex*, 1971, *6*, 215–226.

Harris, A. H., Gilliam, W. J., Findley, J. D., & Brady, J. B. Instrumental conditioning of large magnitude, daily, 12-hour blood pressure elevations in the baboon. *Science*, 1973, *182*, 175–177.

Hefferline, R. F., Keenan, B., & Harford, R. A. Escape and avoidance conditioning in human subjects without their observation of the response. *Science*, 1959, *130*, 1338–1339.

Herd, J. A., Kelleher, R. T., Morse, W. H., & Grose, S. A. Sympathetic and parasympathetic activity during behavioral hypertension in the squirrel monkey. In P. A. Obrist, A. H. Black, J. Brener, & L. V. DiCara (Eds.), *Cardiovascular psychophysiology*. Chicago: Aldine, 1974.

Hnatiow, M., & Lang, P. J. Learned stabilization of cardiac rate. *Psychophysiology*, 1965, *1*, 330–336.

Holroyd, J., Nuechterlein, K., Shapiro, D., & Ward, F. Biofeedback and hypnotizability. In G. D. Burrows, D. R. Collison, & L. Dennerstein (Eds.), *Hypnosis 1979*. New York: Elsevier/North-Holland Biomedical Press, 1979.

Johnson, R. J. Operant reinforcement of an autonomic response. *Dissertation Abstracts*, 1963, *24*, 1255–1256. (Abstract)

Kamiya, J. Operant control of the EEG alpha rhythm and some of its reported effects on consciousness. In C. Tart (Ed.), *Altered states of consciousness*. New York: Wiley, 1969.

Katkin, E. S., & Murray, E. H. Instrumental conditioning of autonomically mediated behavior: Theoretical and methodological issues. *Psychological Bulletin*, 1968, *70*, 52–68.

Keefe, F. J. Conditioning changes in differential skin temperature. *Perceptual and Motor Skills*, 1975, *40*, 283–288.

Keefe, F. J., & Gardner, E. T. Learned control of skin temperature: Effects of short and long-term biofeedback training, *Behavior Therapy*, 1979, *10*, 202–210.

Lang, P. J., Troyer, W. G., Jr., Twentyman, C. T., & Gatchell, R. J. Differential effects of heart rate modification training on college students, older males, and patients with ischemic heart disease *Psychosomatic Medicine*, 1975, *37*, 429–446.

Lang, P. J., & Twentyman, C. T. Learning to control heart rate: Binary versus analogue feedback. *Psychophysiology*, 1974, *11*, 616–629.

Lang, P. J., & Twentyman, C. T. Learning to control heart rate: Effects of varying incentive and criterion of success on task performance. *Psychophysiology*, 1976, *13*, 378–385.

Lisina, M. I. [The role of orientation in the transformation of involuntary into voluntary reactions.] In L. G. Voronin, A. N. Leontiev, A. R. Luria, E. N. Sokolov, & O. S. Vinogradova (Eds.) [*Orienting reflex and exploratory behavior*]. (*Translated from the Russian by Vsevolod Shmelev & Khristan Hanes.*) Washington, D.C.: American Psychological Association, 1965. (Originally published, 1958.)

Lown, B., De Silva, R. A., Reich, P., & Murawski, B. J. Psychophysiologic factors in sudden cardiac death. *The American Journal of Psychiatry*, 1980, *137*, 1325–1335.

Lynch, W. C., Hamma, H., Kohn, S., & Miller, N. E. Instrumental control of peripheral vasomotor responses in children. *Psychophysiology*, 1976, *13*, 219–221.

Manuck, S. B., Levenson, R. W., Hinrichsen, J. J., & Gryll, S. L. Role of feedback in voluntary control of heart rate. *Perceptual and Motor Skills*, 1975, *40*, 747–752.

Maslach C., Marshall, G., & Zimbardo, P. G. Hypnotic control of peripheral skin temperature: A case report. *Psychophysiology*, 1972, *9*, 600–605.

Miller, N. E. Learning of visceral and glandular responses. *Science*, 1969, *163*, 434–445.

Miller, N. E. Applications of learning and biofeedback to psychiatry and medicine. In A. M. Freedman, H. I. Kaplan, & B. J. Sadock (Eds.), *Comprehensive textbook of psychiatry-II*. Baltimore: Williams & Wilkins, 1975.

Miller, N. E., & DiCara, L. Instrumental learning of heart rate changes in curarized rats: Shaping, and specificity to discriminative stimulus. *Journal of Comparative and Physiological Psychology*, 1967, *63*, 12–19.

Miller, N. E., & Dworkin, B. R. Visceral learning: Recent difficulties with curarized rats and significant problems for human research. In P. A. Obrist, A. H. Black, J. Brener, & L. V. DiCara (Eds.), *Cardiovascular psychophysiology*. Chicago: Aldine, 1974.

Obrist, P. A. The cardiovascular–behavioral interaction—As it appears today. *Psychophysiology*, 1976, *13*, 95–107.

Obrist, P. A. *Cardiovascular psychophysiology: A perspective*. New York: Plenum, 1981.

Obrist, P. A., Black, A. H., Brener, J., & DiCara, L. V. (Eds.). *Cardiovascular psychophysiology*. Chicago: Aldine, 1974.

Obrist, P. A., Galosy, R. A., Lawler, J. E., Gaebelein, C. J., Howard, J. L., & Shanks, E. M. Operant conditioning of heart rate: Somatic correlates. *Psychophysiology*, 1975, *12*, 445–455.

Obrist, P. A., Howard, J. L., Lawler, J. E., Galosy, R. A., Meyers, K. A., & Gaebelein, C. J. The cardiac–somatic interaction. In P. A. Obrist, A. H. Black, J. Brener, & L. V. DiCara (Eds.), *Cardiovascular psychophysiology*. Chicago: Aldine, 1974.

Obrist, P. A., Langer, A. W., & Grignolo, A. Pulse propagation time: Relationship in humans to systolic and diastolic blood pressure, heart rate and carotid dP/dt with and without beta-adrenergic blockage. *Psychophysiology*, 1977, *14*, 80–81. (Abstract)

Obrist, P. A., Light, R. C., McCubbin, J. A., Hutcheson, J. S., & Hoffer, J. L. Pulse transit time: Relationship to blood pressure and myocardial performance. *Psychophysiology*, 1979, *16*, 292–301.

Odgen, E., & Shock, N. W. Voluntary hypercirculation. *American Journal of Medical Sciences*, 1939, *198*, 329–342.

Pappas, B. A., DiCara, L. V., & Miller, N. E. Learning of blood pressure responses in the noncurarized rat: Transfer to the curarized state. *Physiology and Behavior*, 1970, *5*, 1029–1032.

Paskowitz, D. A., & Orne, M. T. Visual effects on alpha feedback training. *Science*, 1974, *181*, 360–363.

Patton, H. D. The autonomic nervous system. In T. C. Rugh, H. D. Patton, J. W. Woodbury, & A. L. Towe (Eds.), *Neurophysiology*. Philadelphia: Saunders, 1965.

Pickering, T. G., Brucker, B., Frankel, H. L., Mathias, C. J., Dworkin, B. R., & Miller, N. E. Mechanisms of learned voluntary control of blood pressure in patients with generalised bodily paralysis. In J. Beatty & H. Legewie (Eds.), *Biofeedback and behavior*. New York: Plenum, 1977.

Plumlee, L. A. Operant conditioning of increases in blood pressure. *Psychophysiology*, 1969, *6*, 283–290.

Razran, G. The observable unconscious and the inferable conscious in current Soviet psychophysiology: Interoceptive conditioning, semantic conditioning and the orienting reflex. *Psychological Reviews*, 1961, *68*, 81–147.

Roberts, A., Kewman, D. G., & MacDonald, H. Voluntary control of skin temperature: Unilateral changes using hypnosis and feedback. *Journal of Abnormal Psychology*, 1973, *82*, 163–168.

Roberts, A. H., Schuler, J., Bacon, J. R., Zimmerman, R. L., & Patterson, R. Individual differences and autonomic control: Absorption, hypnotic susceptibility, and the unilateral control of skin temperature. *Journal of Abnormal Psychology*, 1975, *84*, 272–279.

Roberts, L. E. Operant conditioning of autonomic responses: One perspective on the curare experiments. In G. E. Schwartz & D. Shapiro (Eds.), *Consciousness and self-regulation: Advances in research* (Vol. 2.). New York: Plenum, 1978.

Sargent, J. D., Green, E. E., & Walters, E. D. Preliminary report on the use of autogenic feedback training in the treatment of migraine and tension headaches. *Psychosomatic Medicine*, 1973, *35*, 129–135.

Schwartz, G. E. Voluntary control of human cardiovascular integration and differentiation through feedback and reward. *Science*, 1972, *175*, 90–93.

Schwartz, G. E. Toward a theory of voluntary control of response patterns in the cardiovascular system. In P. A. Obrist, A. H. Black, J. Brener, & L. V. DiCara (Eds.), *Cardiovascular psychophysiology*. Chicago: Aldine, 1974.

Shapiro, A. P., & Horn, P. W. Blood pressure, plasma pepsinogen, and behavior in cats subjected to experimental production of anxiety. *Journal of Nervous and Mental Disease*, 1955, *122*, 222–231.

Shapiro, D. [Role of feedback and instructions in the voluntary control of human blood pressure. *Japanese Journal of Biofeedback Research*], 1973, *1*, 2–9. (In Japanese)

Shapiro, D., Crider, A. B., & Tursky, B. Differentiation of an autonomic response through operant reinforcement. *Psychonomic Science,* 1964, *1,* 147–148.

Shapiro, D., Greenstadt, L., Lane, J. D., & Rubinstein, E. Tracking-cuff system for beat-to-beat recording of blood pressure. *Psychophysiology,* 1981, *18,* 129–136.

Shapiro, D., Reeves, J. L., Greenstadt, L., Dolan, P., Cobb, L. F., & Lane, J. D. Blood pressure control using a beat-to-beat tracking-cuff method: Preliminary observations. *Psychophysiology,* 1979, *16,* 175–176. (Abstract)

Shapiro, D., Schwartz, G. E., & Tursky, B. Control of diastolic blood pressure in man by feedback and reinforcement. *Psychophysiology,* 1972, *9,* 296–304.

Shapiro, D., & Surwit, R. S. Behavioral control of psysiological function and disease. In H. Leitenberg (Ed.), *Handbook of behavior modification and behavior therapy.* Englewood Cliffs, N.J.: Prentice-Hall, 1976.

Shapiro, D., Tursky, B., Gershon, E., & Stern, M. Effects of feedback and reinforcement on the control of human systolic blood pressure. *Science,* 1969, *163,* 588–590.

Shapiro, D., Tursky, B., & Schwartz, G. E. Control of blood pressure in man by operant conditioning. *Circulation Research,* 1970, 26–27 (Suppl. No. 1), 27–32. (a)

Shapiro, D., Tursky, B., & Schwartz, G. E. Differentiation of heart rate and systolic blood pressure in man by operant conditioning. *Psychosomatic Medicine,* 1970, *32,* 417–423. (b)

Simonson, E., & Brozek, J. Review: Russian research on arterial hypertension. *Annals of Internal Medicine,* 1959, *50,* 129–193.

Sirota, A. D., Schwartz, G. E., & Shapiro, D. Voluntary control of human heart rate: Effect on reaction to aversive stimulation. *Journal of Abnormal Psychology,* 1974, *83,* 261–267.

Sirota, A. D., Schwartz, G. E., & Shapiro, D. Voluntary control of human heart rate: Effect on reaction to aversive stimulation: A replication and extension. *Journal of Abnormal Psychology,* 1976, *85,* 473–477.

Snyder, C., & Noble, M. E. Operant conditioning of vasoconstriction. *Journal of Experimental Psychology,* 1968, *77,* 263–268.

Sokolow, Y. N. *Perception and the conditioned reflex.* London: Pergamon, 1963.

Stephens, J. H., Harris, A. H., Brady, J. B., & Shaffer, J. W. Psychological and physiological variables associated with large magnitude voluntary heart rate changes. *Psychophysiology,* 1975, *12,* 381–387.

Steptoe, A., & Johnson, D. The control of blood pressure using pulse-wave velocity feedback. *Journal of Psychosomatic Research,* 1976, *20,* 417–424.

Steptoe, A., Mathews, A. M., & Johnson, D. The learned control of differential temperature in the human ear lobes. *Biological Psychology,* 1974, *1,* 237–242.

Steptoe, A., Smulyan, H., & Gribbin, B. Pulse wave velocity and blood pressure: Calibration and applications. *Psychophysiology,* 1976, *13,* 488–493.

Surwit, R. S. Biofeedback: A possible treatment for Raynaud's disease. *Seminars in Psychiatry,* 1973, *5,* 483–490.

Surwit, R. S., Hager, J. L., & Feldman, J. The role of feedback in voluntary control of blood pressure in instructed subjects. *Psychophysiology,* 1977, *14,* 97. (Abstract)

Surwit, R. S., Shapiro, D., & Feld, J. L. Digital temperature autoregulation and associated cardiovascular changes. *Psychophysiology,* 1976, *13,* 242–248.

Taub, E., & Emurian, C. S. Feedback-aided self-regulation of skin temperature with a single feedback locus. I. Acquisition and reversal training. *Biofeedback and Self-Regulation,* 1976, *1,* 147–168.

Trowill, J. A. Instrumental conditioning of the heart rate in the curarized rat. *Journal of Comparative and Physiological Psychology,* 1967, *63,* 7–11.

Wells, D. T. Large magnitude voluntary heart rate changes. *Psychophysiology,* 1973, *10,* 260–269.

Wells, D. T., Feather, B. W., & Headrick, M. W. The effects of immediate feedback upon voluntary control of salivary rate. *Psychophysiology,* 1973, *10,* 501–509.

Whitehead, W. E., Lurie, E., & Blackwell, B. Classical conditioning of decreases in human systolic blood pressure. *Journal of Applied Behavior Analysis,* 1976, *9,* 153–157.

Williams, J. G. L., & Williams, B. Arterial pulse wave velocity as a psychophysiological measure. *Psychosomatic Medicine,* 1965, *5,* 408–413.

Young, L. D., & Blanchard, E. B. Effects of auditory feedback of varying information content on the self control of heart rate. *Psychophysiology,* 1974, *11,* 527–534.

5

Coronary Heart Disease

In the United States during 1970–1979, there was a striking decrease in the death rate due to coronary heart disease (CHD) (see Table 5.1). It is impossible at present to specify with any certainty the reasons for this decline; however, improved methods of acute coronary care, improved means of treating potentially fatal arrythmias, improved surgical treatment approaches, and reductions in behaviors that increase the level of risk factors for CHD are all likely candidates. The final answer will probably never be known, but in all likelihood, all the above factors were involved.

Despite the recent decline, however, the United States continues to have one of the highest CHD death rates in the world. Moreover, CHD continues to be the leading cause of death in the United States, accounting for about 50% more deaths each year than all forms of cancer combined (see Table 5.1). Just as discouraging, the total annual economic cost attributable to cardiovascular diseases, of which the major component is CHD, amounts to over $50 billion in the United States—more than twice that attributable to all forms of cancer. With regard to prevalence and incidence of CHD in the United States population, there is inadequate data with which to define the trends. However, the rate of hospitalization for CHD in the nation's 6700 short-stay hospitals increased by 27% between 1970 and 1975, and for persons aged 45–64—the most productive years of adult life—the rate of hospitalization during this period increased by nearly 40% (DHEW Publication, 1977). Thus, even though the CHD death rate has shown a gratifying decline, it is clear that CHD remains the number one health problem in the United States today.

The basic lesion in CHD is the atheromatous plaque, a mound of tissue built up on the inside of the blood vessel wall and consisting of a core of cholesterol

TABLE 5.1
Death Rates and Percentage Change in Rates Selected Causes of Death
United States, 1970-1975

Cause of death	Rate per 100,000 population[a]		Percentage change
	1970	1975	
All causes	714.3	638.3	−10.6
All cardiovascular disease	350.0	300.3	−14.2
Coronary heart disease	228.1	196.1	−14.0
Stroke	66.3	54.5	−17.8
Hypertensive disease	7.9	5.1	−35.4
Rheumatic heart disease	6.3	4.8	−23.8
All other cardiovascular disease[b]	41.4	39.8	−3.9
All non-cardiovascular disease causes	364.3	338.0	−7.2
Cancer	129.9	130.9	+0.8
Accidents and violence	77.4	70.0	−9.6
Influenza and pneumonia	22.1	16.6	−24.9
Cirrhosis of the liver	14.7	13.8	−6.1
Diabetes	14.1	11.6	−17.7
Chronic obstructive pulmonary disease	13.3	14.3	+7.5
All other	92.8	80.8	−12.9

[a] Age-adjusted to the U.S. population, 1940.
[b] Includes congenital heart disease.
Source: From United States Department of Health, Education and Welfare. The report by the National Heart and Lung Institute Task Force on Arteriosclerosis, December 1977.

and other fats covered by a cap of fibrous scar tissue. As these plaques increase in size and number, they may impede or cut off entirely the blood supply to tissues supplied by these arteries. When the insufficient blood supply is provided by the arteries that supply the heart—the coronary arteries—the result may be ischemia leading to pain or angina pectoris. If the discrepancy between the ability of the artery to supply increased blood flow and the metabolic needs of the tissue is great enough, actual damage is caused to the tissues, resulting in a myocardial infarction, or heart attack. It is not presently known whether blood clot formation, or thrombosis, is also involved in the precipitation of myocardial infarction.

While the complete story remains to be defined, the most widely accepted current theory holds that the initiating mechanism for atheromatous plaque formation involves injury to the endothelial inner lining of the artery, with subsequent accumulation of lipids in the vessel wall and invasion by proliferating smooth muscle cells (Ross & Glomset, 1976). In many instances it is felt that this process of endothelial injury and atheromatous plaque formation begins in childhood and continues into adult life. Then, when the ability of the narrowed coronary artery to deliver blood to meet the needs of the distal myocardial tissue becomes inadequate, as during the experience of strong emotions or exercise, the stage is set for the development of anginal pain or myocardial infarction.

The precise nature of the events necessary for the initiation or progression of atheromatous plaque formation is not known at present. Certain characteristics, known as *risk factors,* have been found in prospective studies of human populations, such as the Framingham Study, to be associated with increased subsequent risk of developing the complications of atherosclerosis, such as heart attack, stroke, and peripheral vascular disease. Until recently, the three main established risk factors were (*a*) high levels of blood cholesterol, particularly that associated with low-density lipoproteins (LDL), (*b*) high blood pressure, and (*c*) cigarette smoking (Kannel, McGee, & Gordon, 1976). These traditional risk factors, however, do not allow us to predict which individuals will develop coronary disease and appear to account for no more than 50% of the variance in CHD rates (Keys, 1966). It is clear, therefore, that other risk factors remain to be identified before we can achieve an adequate understanding of the etiology and pathogenesis of CHD.

In the search for these additional risk factors, there has been a steadily increasing recognition of the role of psychosocial and behavioral characteristics that also appear to place individuals at increased risk of developing CHD. There is now extensive evidence that stressful life events may be playing a role in the precipitation of acute clinical CHD events. The role of the social milieu, particularly in terms of the availability of support networks, also appears important in moderating the impact of life events. Finally, a specific behavior pattern, the Type A (or coronary-prone) behavior pattern, has been shown in a body of extensive and wide-ranging research (Dembroski, Weiss, Shields, Haynes, & Feinleib, 1978) to be a risk factor whose contribution to "risk [of CHD] is over and above that imposed by age, systolic blood pressure, serum cholesterol and smoking and [which] appears to be of the same order of magnitude as the relative risk associated with any of these other factors [NHLBI, 1978]." Thus, Type A behavior pattern is now recognized as an established risk factor, along with high blood pressure, high cholesterol, and cigarette smoking.

In this chapter we shall review the evidence suggesting the involvement of these psychosocial and behavioral factors in the etiology and pathogenesis of CHD. In addition we shall consider the role of behavioral factors in the prevention, treatment, and rehabilitation of CHD.

ETIOLOGY AND PATHOGENESIS

Stressful Life Events and Social Supports

In addition to the well-documented contribution to increased risk of CHD associated with such traditional risk factors as high blood pressure, high levels of serum cholesterol and cigarette smoking, evidence is accumulating that psychological, behavioral, and sociocultural factors are also important in the etiology and pathogenesis of CHD (Jenkins, 1971, 1976). There is evidence that stressful life events are likely to be followed by a wide variety of illnesses, including clinical CHD events. The impact of stressful life events appears to be modulated by the presence or absence of social support networks in the individual's current environment.

With regard to the role of stressful life events, it has been shown that the risk of CHD increases with major changes in place of residence (Syme, Borhani, & Buechley, 1965; Syme, Hyman, & Enterline, 1964), major changes in occupation (Kaplan, Cassel, Tyroler, Cornoni, Kleinbaum, & Hames, 1971; Shekelle, Ostfeld, & Paul, 1969), and the occurence of discrepancies between the culture of upbringing and current sociocultural situation (Medalie, Kahn, Neufeld, Riss, Goldbourt, Perlstein, & Oron, 1973). While it is not clear at present whether this increase in risk occurs as a result of mobility per se or as a result of personal characteristics that predispose certain individuals to become mobile, there is at least one study (Tyroler & Cassel, 1964) showing increased CHD rates among persons who were not mobile but who experienced changes in the situation in which they lived. Another theme in the life change literature addresses the role of various kinds of losses that may influence health (Rahe, 1972). Despite problems with retrospective designs in earlier work, a number of studies are now available in which these problems are not at issue. Thus, a number of studies have shown an increased rate of CHD among widows and widowers shortly after the death of their spouses, and other studies have shown increases in blood pressure among those recently unemployed (Dohrenwend & Dohrenwend, 1974).

The evidence cited in the preceding paragraph suggests some involvement of stressful life events in the long-term accumulation of processes involved in the development of the atheromatous plaque and/or the precipitation of acute CHD events. In addition to this evidence, other data, albeit anecdotal, suggest a linkage between single traumatic events and almost immediate cardiac death. Engel (1971) collected and analyzed 170 accounts from newspapers and other sources of sudden death occurring in the setting of extreme emotional arousal. He notes that more than half of these events are concerned with the loss or threatened loss of important others in the victim's life. A 61-year-old woman collapsed immediately upon hearing of her sister's sudden death and died shortly afterward of cardiac arrest. A 40-year-old father slumped dead as he held the head of his son lying injured in the street beside his motorcycle. Other types of loss also may be capable of precipitating sudden cardiac death. Engel reports the case of a 52-year-old college president who prided himself on his support of black students and who "died when a group of black students occupied the administration building." Another case involved a "57 year old state legislator [who] died 48 hours after being convicted of bribery and sentenced to prison." Loss of others or of self-esteem were not the only events found associated with sudden cardiac death; Engel (1971) also found instances of sudden death following positive life events—for example, the 60-year-old prisoner who "collapsed and died when he returned home to his family after serving a 15-year sentence," or the 55-year-old man and his 88-year-old father who both died suddenly on meeting after a 20-year separation.

It is most likely that such instances of sudden death in the setting of extreme emotional excitement occur in persons with preexisting CHD (Spain, Brodess, & Mohr, 1960). The most likely physiological mechanism accounting for these deaths would appear to involve activation of the defense reaction (see Chapter 3), with its sudden release of catecholamines and attendant acutely increased demands for cardiac work. While such acute changes are well tolerated in the healthy individual, in the setting of preexisting coronary atherosclerosis, it is likely that the acute increase in work load on the heart could precipitate fatal myocardial infarction, while the increased catecholamines could also precipitate fatal arrythmias, particularly in ischemic myocardial tissue.

While the kind of evidence cited here linking stressful life events with increased rates of clinical CHD events is provocative, it is clear that other aspects of the social milieu and the psychobehavioral makeup of the person play an important role in moderating the impact of life events upon health. One characteristic of the individual that is important in this regard is the tendency to behave in a manner that has come to be described as Type A, and we shall review the evidence linking Type A behavior pattern and CHD in some detail later in this chapter. First, however, we will conclude our discussion of the impact of the environment on the risk of CHD by considering the role of social support networks in moderating the impact of stressful life events. Social support is defined as information available to the individual leading to beliefs in three areas (Cobb, 1976):

1. Information leading to the belief that one is loved and cared for
2. Information leading to the belief that one is esteemed and valued by other individuals or groups
3. Information leading to the belief that one belongs to a network of communication and mutual obligation

Cobb (1976) cites extensive evidence documenting a relatively smaller negative effect of life change on health among persons with high levels of social support compared to persons with low levels of social support, even when exposed to the same life events. There is also evidence suggesting that low levels of social support exert an adverse effect upon CHD risk, whereas high levels of social support appear protective against CHD risk.

In a 9-year follow-up study of 6928 persons, Berkman and Syme (1979) found an increased mortality rate among persons previously identified as having fewer friends and contacts with other persons. This relationship was linear and independent of health status at baseline as well as of such other risk factors as obesity, cigarette smoking, physical inactivity, and other health habits. These findings suggest that persons without the kinds of social support that would be provided by more frequent ties between people are at greater risk of CHD.

In their studies of Japanese migrants to Hawaii and California, Marmot and Syme (1976) observed an increased rate of CHD among those living in California but were unable to account for this in terms of differences in diet, age, serum cholesterol, blood pressure, or cigarette smoking. However, what did distinguish between groups of Japanese living in California with high versus low CHD rates was the degree to which they had retained traditional Japanese life-styles and associations. Figure 5.1 shows that among those who had a traditional Japanese upbringing and whose dentist or physician ("ethnicity of professional") was Japanese, the CHD rate was less than one-fifth that observed among Japanese Californians with neither a traditional upbringing nor a Japanese dentist or physician. Interestingly, among those with *either* a traditional upbringing or a Japanese dentist or physician, the CHD rate was intermediate. The most traditional group had CHD rates that were as low as

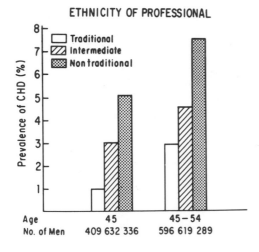

FIGURE 5.1. CHD rates of Japanese migrants living in Hawaii and California with and without traditional Japanese upbringing. [From M. G. Marmot & S. L. Syme. Acculturation and coronary heart disease in Japanese-Americans. *American Journal of Epidemiology,* 1976, *104,* 242.]

those observed in Japan. Marmot and Syme (1976) cited evidence that traditional Japanese maintain more close and intimate ties with family and friends and interpreted the lower CHD rate among traditional Japanese Americans as evidence "that a stable society whose members enjoy the support of their fellows in closely knit groups may protect against the forms of social stress that may lead to CHD [p. 245]." As will be noted later when we consider the evidence relating to the Type A behavior pattern, there may be alternative explanations for the low CHD rates among Japanese Americans. Nevertheless, these findings are at least supportive of the hypothesis that strong social support networks are protective against CHD risk and that this effect is independent of the traditional risk factors of high blood pressure, high cholesterol, and cigarette smoking.

The Type A Behavior Pattern

As was noted earlier, the Type A behavior pattern is the psychobehavioral characteristic with the strongest and most extensive evidence indicating that it plays a role in the etiology and pathogenesis of CHD. The National Heart, Lung and Blood Institute in 1978 convened a panel of distinguished behavioral and biomedical scientists to review the evidence (Dembroski, Weiss, Shields, Haynes, & Feinleib, 1978) linking Type A behavior pattern with increased CHD risk (NHLBI, 1978). One of the conclusions reached was that Type A is an independent risk factor for CHD. Thus, in the future, Type A behavior pattern should be included along with high blood pressure, high levels of serum cholesterol, and cigarette smoking in any listing of "established" CHD risk factors. In the discussion that follows, we shall review (a) the origins of the Type A behavior pattern, (b) how it is assessed, (c) the evidence linking it with various CHD manifestations, and (d) the possible mechanisms mediating the observed association with CHD.

Origins of the Type A Behavior Pattern

Physicians and psychologists have long been aware that certain features have characterized many patients with coronary disease. For example, the German physician Von Dusch (1868) observed that individuals with loud speech and excessive work habits were predisposed to develop CHD. In 1897, Sir William Osler noted "in the worry and strain of modern life, arterial degeneration is not only very common but develops at a relatively early age. For this, I believe that the high pressure at which men live, and the habit of working the machine to its maximum capacity are responsible [for coronary disease]." Writing later in the *Lancet,* he went on to suggest that the typical coronary patient was "not the delicate neurotic" but "the *robust,* the *vigorous* in mind and body, the *keen* and *ambitious* man, the indicator of whose engine is always at *full speed ahead* [Osler, 1910; emphasis added]"

More systematic later reports (Arlow, 1945; Dunbar, 1943; Kemple, 1945; Menninger & Menninger, 1936) reemphasized various psychobehavioral characteristics of coronary patients. Often mentioned were such features as extreme competitiveness, hostility, chronic tension, and overwork. Stuart Wolfe (1969) compared the coronary patient to Sisyphus, the mythological king of Corinth who, when condemned to Hades, was compelled endlessly to push a huge stone up the side of a hill. Each time he approached the top, the stone would roll down again, requiring him to do more and more work without ever experiencing a feeling of accomplishment. Such an analogy underscores the basic lack of satisfaction and sense of fulfillment that the coronary patient often experiences, despite such overt indications of success as wealth, fame, or status.

In the 1950s, Friedman and Rosenman (1959), two cardiologists at the Harold Bruhn Institute at Mt. Zion Hospital in San Francisco, combined these characteristics with several new features in their formulation of the Type A behavior pattern. This pattern was defined as an "action-emotion complex" exhibited by an individual who is engaged in a relatively chronic and excessive struggle to obtain an unlimited number of poorly defined things from his environment in the shortest period of time and, if necessary, against the opposing efforts of others. This struggle is reflected in activity designed to do more in less time, often at the expense of others.

David Jenkins (1971) has described the Type A individual in the following manner:

> The coronary-prone behavior pattern is considered to be an overt behavioral syndrome or style of living characterized by *extremes* of competitiveness, striving for achievement, aggressiveness (sometimes stringently repressed), haste, impatience, restlessness, hyperalertness, explosiveness of speech, tenseness of facial musculature and feelings of being under the pressure of time and under the challenge of responsibility. Persons having this pattern are often so deeply committed to their vocation or profession that other aspects of their lives are relatively neglected. Not all aspects of this syndrome or pattern need be present for a person to be classified as possessing it. The pattern is neither a personality trait nor a standard reaction of a characterologically predisposed person to a situation which challenges him. Different kinds of situations evoke maximal reaction from different persons [p. 312].

People who exhibit a preponderance of these Type A characteristics are classified as Type A. The converse, the Type B behavior pattern, is characterized by a relative absence of these characteristics.

The distinction between the conceptualization underlying the research on Type A behavior pattern and the primary focus upon intrapsychic personality factors in traditional psychosomatic medicine approaches to the study of etiology and pathogenesis was highlighted at the Timberline Conference on Psychophysiologic Aspects of Cardiovascular Disease in 1964. Rosenman's presentation of the then available data pertaining to the relationship between Type A behavior and coronary disease was strongly criticized as inadequate because it did not attempt to define the important traits in a personality that could be related to disease processes (Timberline Conference, 1964). Rosenman's response to these criticisms was quite consistent with behavioral medicine's focus on overt, observable behavior:

> We have not concerned ourselves with factors of motivation but only with determining the presence or absence of the *overt* pattern A, and I suspect that [those objecting to absence of concern with personality traits] are upset at this as well as our seeming oversimplification of inexact factors that are difficult to assess and even more difficult to quantitate [however] it is possible . . . to study different aspects of men that are tall and men that are short . . . without determining why they are tall or short . . . [Timberline Conference, 1964].

Assessment of the Type A Behavior Pattern

There are two widely accepted approaches for determining the presence of the Type A behavior pattern: a structured behavioral interview (Rosenman, Friedman, Straus, Wurm, Kositchek, Hahn, & Werthessen, 1964) and a self-administered questionnaire, the Jenkins Activity Survey for Health Prediction (JAS) (Jenkins, Rosenman, & Friedman, 1967). The structured interview is designed to present the individual with a series of questions in order to elicit Type A behaviors. Assessment of the pattern is based as much on the style as the content of the response. The JAS, on the other hand, is an objective, computer-scored questionnaire that is based solely upon response content. The JAS shows about 65–70% classification agreement with the structured interview but approaches 90% at the extreme ends of the distribution.

Structured Interview. The classification of individuals as Type A or Type B is usually determined by clinical judgments based upon a series of specific questions. These questions are designed to elicit a particular *style* of response that is often displayed by Type A individuals, as well as to determine data regarding the individual's typical behavior based on self-reported attitudes and practices.

The subject is asked approximately 20–25 questions dealing with feelings of ambition and competitiveness, past history of feelings of anger, sense of time urgency and impatience, and current feelings of irritation and frustration. The manner in which the interview is conducted attempts to create a situation whereby Type A behaviors can be observed. For example, the interviewer purposely interrupts the subject to elicit anger, asks questions rapidly to encourage a quick response, and slows the question, "stumbling" over words, to facilitate an interruption on the part of the respondent. In this way, assessment of the Type A behavior pattern depends more on *overt behavior* than on the self-reported habitual behaviors of the subject.

The Type A pattern may be independently classified along several different behavioral dimensions. For example, Type A individuals may speak with a rapid, staccato speech style, frequently emphasizing key words; they may display impatience by attempting to hurry the interviewer by displaying anticipatory nods or by such verbalizations as "yes" or "ahem"; they may demonstrate hostility by their frequent use of profanity or by their signs of irritability or annoyance.

The Type A behavior pattern is best identified by observing the individual in action. It is displayed in speech style, motoric gestures and movements, and style of interaction, as well as the individual's orientation to work and quality of

TABLE 5.2
Features of Type A and Type B Individuals

Type A behavior pattern	Type B behavior pattern
1. A general expression of vigor and energy, alertness and confidence	1. A general expression of relaxation, calm and quiet attentiveness
2. A firm handshake and brisk walking pace	2. A gentle handshake and a moderate to slow walking pace
3. Loud and/or vigorous voice	3. A mellow voice usually low in volume
4. Terse speech, abbreviated responses	4. Lengthy, rambling responses
5. Clipped speech (a failure to pronounce the ending sounds of words)	5. No evidence of clipped speech
6. Rapid speech and acceleration of speech at the end of a longer sentence	6. Slow to moderate pacing of verbal responses. No acceleration at the end of a sentence
7. Explosive speech (speech punctuated with certain words spoken emphatically and this is established as the speaker's general pattern) that may contain swear words	7. Minimum inflection in general speech, almost a monotone with no explosive quality
8. Interrupting by frequent rapid responses given before another speaker has completed his question or statement	8. Rarely interrupts another speaker

(*continued*)

TABLE 5.2 (*Continued*)

Type A behavior pattern	Type B behavior pattern
9. Speech hurrying in the form of saying "yes, yes," or "mm, mm," or "right, right," or by nodding his head in assent while another person speaks	9. No speech hurrying
10. Vehement reactions to questions relating to impedance of time-progress (i.e., driving slowly, waiting in lines)	10. No vehement reactions to questions related to impedance of making progress with utilization of time
11. Use of clenched fist or pointing his finger at you to emphasize his verbalization	11. Never uses the clenched fist or the pointing finger gesture to emphasize his speech
12. Frequent sighing especially related to questions about his work. It is important to differentiate this from the sighs of a depressed person	12. Rarely sighs unless he is "hyperventilating" and showing nervous anxiety
13. Hostility directed at the interviewer or at the topics of the interview	13. Hostility is rarely, if ever, observed
14. Frequent, abrupt and emphatic one-word responses to your questions (i.e., Yes! Never! Definitely! Absolutely!)	14. An absence of emphatic, one-word responses

Source: From J. A. Blumenthal, & R. B. Williams. In P. Boudewyns & F. Keefe (Eds.), *Behavioral Medicine for the primary care physician.* Addison-Wesley, in press.

interpersonal relationships. Table 5.2 summarizes the outstanding features of both Type A and Type B individuals. The following case examples demonstrate the two contrasting behavioral styles:

Case #1: Mr. A is a 43-year-old building contractor. He arrives for his appointment 15 min early and paces in the waiting room as he anxiously awaits his physician's arrival. He can be heard to be engaging in what can only be described as "tuneless humming." When his doctor is late, he becomes visibly irritated and impatient, often displaying overt frustration and hostility. ("I'm busy, too—in my business if I'm late I would lose a customer!") His speech style is rapid, loud, and clipped. He frequently emphasizes certain key words by increasing his speech volume or by gesturing with his hands. While he appears superficially to be intensely involved in the conversation, sometimes he does not really seem to be listening. He asks many questions, and despite his acknowledgment that "you're the doctor," he seems intent upon being in control of the situation. He is extremely dedicated to his work, and his family life seems to be of secondary importance. While he appears extraverted and congenial, he is difficult to get to know and seems superficial in his relations. He is extremely concerned about his condition and gives the impression that he is the only person who ever experienced his symptoms.

The Type B individual is more relaxed and easygoing. His speech style is slow and regular. He does not appear hostile, impatient, or competitive and seems calm, satisfied, and content.

Case #2: Mr. B is a 53-year-old accountant. He may be somewhat nervous but is not impatient or restless. He waits calmly for his turn and does not appear rushed or pressured. He seems to reflect on his thoughts before speaking and listens attentively without interrupting or anticipating the doctor's reply. He presents his symptoms carefully and seems to exhibit a basic trust in his physician. He listens attentively and displays a calm, pleasant disposition.

Jenkins Activity Survey (JAS). In order to provide an objective measure of the Type A behavior pattern, the JAS was developed and standardized on a sample of over 3000 employed males participating in the Western Collaborative Group Study (WCGS). Items that discriminated between subjects judged to be Type A and those judged to be Type B were selected for inclusion in the Type A subscale. The validity of the JAS is based upon agreement between its scores and ratings made by the structured interview and upon its ability to predict the incidence and prevalence of CHD. Further refinement of the JAS has yielded three additional factor-analytically derived subscales, called speed and impatience, job involvement, and hard driving. Typical questions include:

1. Has your spouse or some friend ever told you that you eat too fast? Type A subjects indicate "Yes, often," whereas Type B subjects indicate "No, no one has told me this."
2. When you listen to someone talking and this person takes too long to come to the point, do you feel like hurrying him along? Type A subjects indicate "Frequently," whereas Type B subjects indicate "Almost never."
3. How is your temper nowadays? Type A subjects indicate "Fiery, hard to control" or "Strong but controllable," whereas Type B subjects indicate "I almost never get angry."
4. Do you ever set deadlines or quotas for yourself at work or at home? Type A subjects respond "Yes, once a week or more often," whereas Type B subjects usually respond "No."

The JAS is standardized to have a mean of 0.0 and a standard deviation of 10.0. Scores in the positive direction denote Type A characteristics, while scores in the negative direction indicate Type B behavior. The comparative validity and utility of the JAS have been discussed in detail elsewhere (Jenkins, 1978). The stylistic features of the Type A behavior pattern are best observed *in vivo;* questionnaire data may be spuriously affected by response bias or inaccurate self-reports. Nevertheless, available evidence indicates that the Type A behavior pattern as assessed by the JAS is related to significantly greater incidence and prevalence of CHD, including myocardial infarction (MI), recurring MI, and coronary atherosclerosis. The next section will consider in greater detail the evidence relating Type A to the clinical manifestations of CHD.

While assessment using either the structured interview or the JAS has identified characteristics that are reliably predictive of increased CHD risk, only a small proportion of Type A individuals go on to develop clinically apparent CHD over follow-up periods of up to 8.5 years. This suggests that within the Type A population there are other characteristics—psychological, behavioral, physiological, and/or neurohumoral—remaining to be identified that could serve to subgroup further the heterogeneous Type A population into subgroups that are more homogeneous with regard to risk of CHD. Eventually, assessment of these more prognostically relevant subcomponents of the global Type A pattern will undoubtedly replace both the structured interview and the JAS. At that point, it is likely that we shall be in a position to explain considerably more than 50% of the variance in CHD incidence.

Association of Type A and Coronary Disease

The Western Collaborative Group Study (WCGS) is the landmark study in the Type A literature. Previously, Rosenman and Friedman reported that Type A men and women had four to seven times the rate of CHD compared to their Type B counterparts in two retrospective studies (Friedman & Rosenman, 1959; Rosenman & Friedman, 1961). The WCGS project was initiated in 1960–1961 as a *prospective,* epidemiologic study of the incidence of coronary disease in 3524 men aged 39–59 years at intake and employed in 11 participating companies in California. At the beginning of the study, subjects underwent extensive medical evaluation in which a complete medical history was obtained, blood studies and other laboratory tests including electrocardiograms (EKGs) were performed, and the structured Type A behavioral interview was administered. Initially, 113 men were found to have manifest CHD; of these, 80 men, or almost 71%, were judged to be Type A (Rosenman *et al.,* 1964). A remaining sample of 3154 subjects were diagnosed as being free from disease and were subsequently followed annually for a mean period of 8.5 years. The results of the study were published in the *Journal of the American Medical Association* (Rosenman, Brand, Jenkins, Friedman, Straus, & Wurm, 1975) and are summarized in Figure 5.2.

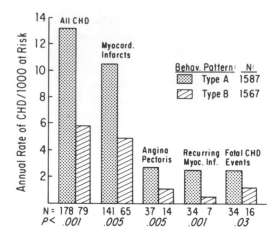

FIGURE 5.2. CHD incidence for all subjects during 8½ year follow-up according to behavior pattern. [From Friedman, M., & Rosenman, R. H. *Annals of Clinical Research*, 1971, 3, 305.]

Of the 257 men that developed CHD during this interval, 178 were classified as Type A, while only 79 were considered Type B. Thus, the Type A subjects exhibited 2.25 times the rate of new CHD compared to their Type B counterparts. A statistical adjustment procedure (Brand, 1978) using the multiple logistic model to control for differences in age, serum cholesterol, systolic blood pressure, and smoking reduced the relative risk to approximately 1.97. In addition, it should be noted that recurring MIs were observed in 41 subjects, 34 of whom were initially classified as Type A. This fivefold greater rate of recurrent MIs was highly significant for both the 39–49 and 50–59 age groups.

These findings were based on behavior pattern classification using the structured interview. At the 1965 annual reexamination of the WCGS group, 2946 men (or 92% of the remaining sample) completed the 1965 version of the JAS. Jenkins, Rosenman, and Zyzanski (1974) found that those men who developed CHD after testing ($N = 120$) scored significantly higher on the Type A scale than did a random sample of controls ($N = 524$).

In addition, there was a significant *linear* relationship between Type A scores and the risk of new coronary disease: the higher the Type A score, the greater the CHD risk. In sum, although the JAS Type A scale does not classify subjects in the same way as the structured interview (correlations are reported between .40 and .80), the Type A scale has been shown to be a significant predictor of CHD events, albeit not as good as the interview assessment. Moreover, numerous retrospective studies from a variety of investigative teams have documented a positive association between the JAS Type A scale and clinical coronary events, including an even stronger relationship between Type A and risk of recurrent MI. The JAS has been translated into other languages, including French, Flemish, German, Polish, and Japanese, and several reports are now available documenting an association between Type A scores on the JAS and increased prevalence of coronary disease in Europe. For more detailed information, the interested reader is referred to several excellent reviews (Dembroski, Weiss, & Shields, 1978; Glass, 1977; Jenkins, 1976).

In addition to studies that examine the relation between the Type A behavior pattern and the incidence and prevalence of MI, several studies have now been published reporting a relationship between Type A and coronary atherosclerosis. By 1966, 51 of 82 subjects who had died during the WCGS were examined at autopsy for evidence of occlusions of the coronary arteries. Friedman, Rosenman, Straus, Wurm, and Kositchek (1968) reported that significantly more atherosclerosis was found in men judged to have been Type A than was found in men judged to have been Type B. Of the 30 subjects who were diagnosed as having severe artery disease, 26 were classified as Type A.

These findings were extended in a study of patients referred to Duke University Medical Center for diagnostic coronary angiography. Patients underwent a routine cardiology workup followed by coronary angiography. Psychological data, including information from the structured Type A interview, were obtained after the angiography but before the results of the procedure were known. Angiograms were interpreted by a panel of three cardiologists experienced in interpreting angiographic films, using a point system for grading the severity of stenosis in each of the four major vessels. Patients exhibiting stenosis of 75% or greater in any vessel were considered to have significant disease. Medical and psychological data were not exchanged until the completion of the study.

The initial report presented data from 80 men and 62 women (Blumenthal, Williams, Kong, Schanberg, & Thompson, 1978) showing that, while 44% of the patients with mild coronary occlusions were classified as Type A by the interview, 69% of those with moderate occlusion were judged to be Type A and 93% of all patients with severe disease were assessed as being Type A (see Figure 5.3). This increased proportion of Type As in the group with more severe atherosclerosis remained highly significant even with adjustment for age, sex, blood pressure, serum cholesterol, and history of cigarette smoking.

This study has now been extended to include a new sample of 307 men and 117 women, all of whom were referred to Duke for coronary angiography because of suspected coronary artery disease. The latest results (Williams, Haney, Lee, Kong, Blumenthal, & Whalen, 1980) indicate that 71% of the 319 patients who were judged to be Type A on the basis of the interview were found to have a significant coronary atherosclerosis, whereas only 56% of the 105 non-Type A had significant disease. It should be noted that this sample consisted of a sizable proportion of female subjects, and the relationship between Type A and extent of coronary atherosclerosis was at least as strong for the women as for the men. Two other research groups have also found a significant association between increased levels of coronary atherosclerosis and the Type A behavior pattern using both the structured interview (Frank, Heller, Kornfeld, Sporn, & Weiss, 1978) and the JAS (Zyzanski, Jenkins, Ryan, Flessas, & Everist, 1976). A third group (Dimsdale, Hackett, Hutter, Block, & Catanzano, 1978) failed to confirm this association using either the JAS or the structured interview. The reasons for this discrepancy are unclear at present. Perhaps they result from differences among the study populations with regard to some unassessed characteristic. In ongoing studies at Duke, it is found that, while the proportions of Type As and Type Bs may not differ that markedly among groups with only mild to moderate lesions, among patients with very severe coronary atherosclerosis, fewer than 10% are Type Bs. It appears, therefore, that, although more research is clearly indicated (particularly as noninvasive means of studying coronary anatomy in healthy subjects becomes available), the weight of current evidence suggests that the Type A behavior pattern is involved in the process of atherogenesis as well as in the precipitation of acute events.

One of the most encouraging new directions for Type A research has been the study of relationships between behavioral subcomponents of the Type A pattern and various manifestations of CHD. For example, Matthews, Glass, Rosenman, and Bortner (1977) analyzed the WCGS data in an effort to identify a subset of factors that were related to CHD. Two factors, competitive drive and impatience, were associated with subsequent occurrence of coronary disease. Examination of item content revealed that potential for hostility and irritability were especially prominent. Examination of the Duke sample undergoing coronary catheterization confirms the importance of the hostility component of Type A (Williams *et al.*, 1980). The Cook and Medley (1954) hostility

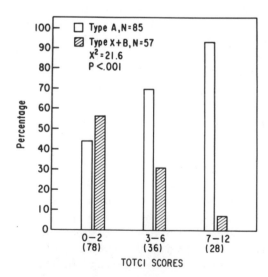

FIGURE 5.3. Type A behavior pattern as function of severity of coronary atherosclerosis. [From J. A. Blumenthal, R. B. Williams, Y. Kong, S. M. Schanberg, & L. W. Thompson. Type A behavior pattern and coronary atherosclerosis. *Circulation*, 1979, 58, 637.]

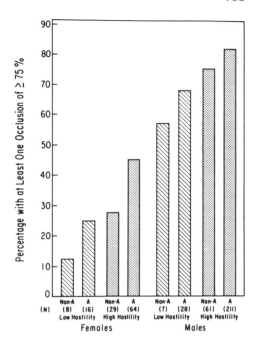

FIGURE 5.4. Relation of Type A behavior pattern, hostility, and gender to presence of significant coronary occlusions. [From R. B. Williams, T. L. Haney, K. L. Lee, Y. Kong, J. A. Blumenthal, & R. E. Whalen. Type A behavior, hostility and coronary atherosclerosis, *Psychosomatic Medicine*, 1980, 42, 545.]

scale of the Minnesota Multiphasic Personality Inventory (MMPI)—a standard instrument used for psychometric assessment—was administered to all subjects. Patients classified as Type A scored significantly higher on hostility than patients classified as non-Type A. Only 48% of the sample scoring less than or equal to 10 on the hostility scale were found to have significant disease, whereas 70% of the subjects who obtained scores greater than 10 had significant disease. Statistical analysis revealed that hostility was significantly related to coronary atherosclerosis, independent of gender or behavior pattern classification. Figure 5.4 shows the striking relationship between Type A, hostility, and gender. There is an observed linear increment of risk ranging from the low-risk group (low hostile, non-Type A women), of whom 12.5% had significant disease, to the highest risk group (Type A, hostile males), of whom 82% had significant occlusions of at least one artery. Among the 117 women in this sample, there is almost a fourfold greater likelihood of having a significant lesion when the high hostile, Type A group is compared to the low hostile, non-Type A group.

This apparent protective effect associated with very low scores on the hostility scale may provide an alternative explanation of the Marmot and Syme's (1976) finding (discussed earlier) of reduced CHD rates among Japanese in California who adhere to traditional Japanese culture. They interpreted that protective effect as related to increased levels of social support in traditional

Japanese culture. It appears equally likely, however, that traditional Japanese, with their high investment in a group identity and close ties with family and friends, would be most unlikely to endorse more than 10 items on the Cook and Medley (1954) hostility scale, especially when it is recalled that endorsement of these items generally reflects "dislike for and distrust of people [p. 417]." Thus, the low CHD rates among Japanese Californians with a traditional Japanese cultural orientation may be due to the extremely low levels of hostility that would be expected among persons with such a cultural orientation.

Psychophysiological Mechanisms Underlying the Association between Type A and CHD

As previously noted, the Type A behavior pattern has been found to be associated not only with an increased incidence of acute CHD clinical events (MI and sudden death) but also with increased levels of the underlying pathological lesion, coronary atherosclerosis. These associations suggest the existence of mechanisms that link psychobehavioral processes—most likely via central nervous system (CNS) mediation—with those processes involved in the formation of the atherosclerotic plaque, as well as with the acute initiation of clinical events. Extensive laboratory, clinical, and epidemiologic evidence exists that suggests that such mechanisms involve (a) hormonal and lipid responses in association with varying behavioral states, and (b) physiological responses in association with varying behavioral states.

A number of studies by Friedman, Rosenman, and co-workers have shown that extreme Type A persons exhibit exaggerated hormonal and lipid responses to various behavioral challenges. Type A subjects have generally been found to have higher levels of serum cholesterol than their Type B counterparts, both prior to the emergence of clinically evident CHD (Friedman, Byers, Rosenman, & Elevitch, 1970) and after the clinical stage is reached (Blumenthal et al., 1978). Despite increased serum levels of adrenocorticotrophic hormone (ACTH) (Friedman, Byers, & Rosenman, 1972), Type A persons show a subnormal cortisol response to administration of exogenous ACTH (Friedman, 1969). This suggests that among Type A persons frequent and chronic arousal responses have resulted in a depletion of adrenal cortical reserves. Similarly, serum growth hormone levels are reduced among Type A subjects, both before and following challenge with arginine (Friedman, Byers, Rosenman, & Newman, 1971). With regard to sympathetic nervous system function, Type A subjects have been found both to excrete increased amounts of norepinephrine during a typical work day (Friedman, St. George, & Byers, 1960) and to show elevated serum norepinephrine levels during a challenging competitive task (Friedman, Byers, Diament, & Rosenman, 1975).

There is now a rapidly growing body of research from several laboratories concerned with identifying differences in psychophysiological response between Type A and Type B individuals. This research is a logical extension of the earlier work cited here with regard to enhanced excretion or secretion of catecholamines or their metabolites among Type A subjects. If it can be shown that Type A individuals reliably exhibit excessive sympathetic arousal in response to specific challenge, an important step will have been taken toward defining the mechanisms through which behavior plays a role in the pathogenic processes in CHD (Williams, Friedman, Glass, Herd, & Schneiderman, 1978).

Dembroski, MacDougall, Shields, Petitto, and Lushene (1978) studied the physiological responses of 50 Type A and Type B subjects who were challenged to respond rapidly and accurately on three tasks involving either perceptual-motor or cognitive skills. In general, it was found that Type A subjects showed significantly greater cardiovascular changes indicative of sympathetic nervous system arousal than did Type B subjects. In addition, it was found that increased levels of hostility or competitiveness during the structured interview were predictive of heightened physiological responses during the tasks. Utilizing a similar set of challenging experimental tasks, Manuck, Craft, and Gold (1978) found Type A males to show greater systolic blood pressure elevations during task performance in comparison to Type B males. Interestingly, this effect was not found among the females studied.

In an extension of earlier work, Dembroski, MacDougall, Herd, and Shields (1978) subjected Type A and Type B subjects to the cold pressor test and a reaction time task under conditions of both high and low challenge. They found that Type A subjects were more physiologically responsive overall, though this effect was most pronounced under high-challenge conditions. When the subjects were also categorized with regard to levels of hostility and competitiveness, it was found that, in contrast to Type B subjects, Type A subjects who also displayed high levels of hostility or competitiveness were hyperresponsive physiologically to both low- and high-challenge instructions during the cold pressor and reaction time tasks. In addition to the differential effect of hostility and competitiveness on the physiological responses of Type A as compared to Type B subjects demonstrated in this study, Scherwitz, Berton, and Leventhal (1978) found that high levels of self-involvement (measured as the simple frequency of use of personal pronouns during the structured interview) were related to elevated levels of cardiovascular response across a wide variety of experimental tasks among Type A but not Type B subjects.

In addition to these empirical studies, we have proposed both in Chapter 3 and elsewhere (Williams, 1975) that both alpha-adrenergically mediated vasoconstrictor responses during sensory intake, or vigilance behaviors and beta-adrenergically mediated cardiac output responses during mental work or emergency situations are two potential mechanisms whereby physiological responding during qualitatively different behavioral states contribute both to the process of atherogenesis and to the precipitation of acute clinical events. Ongoing studies have recently produced evidence which supports this hypothesis: Whether behavior pattern is assessed by the JAS or the Structured Interview, Type A male undergraduates show a significantly larger increase in forearm blood flow (an index of muscle blood flow—see Chapter 2) and a larger increase in plasma epinephrine and cortisol than do Type Bs during a challenging mental arithmetic task (Williams *et al.*, 1981; Note 3).

The chronic overactivity of neuroendocrine, lipid metabolism, and physiological response systems suggested in Type A persons by the above considerations could play a role in the atherosclerotic process by promoting episodes of "endothelial injury," postulated by Ross and Glomset (1976) to be the initiating event in atherogenesis. In addition, the excessive sympathetic stimulation could be important in the precipitation of acute events by increasing myocardial oxygen needs, as well as by direct effects on cardiac electrical impulse conduction leading to potentially fatal arrythmias. Extensive research efforts are now being mounted to test these hypotheses. As we define with greater precision not only differences in psychophysiological and neuroendocrine responsivity *between* As and Bs, but also begin to identify subgroups *within* the Type A population who are hyperresponsive compared to other Type As, it is likely that the accuracy of our prognostic attempts will show considerable improvement.

In summary, we can now state with some assurance that it is possible to identify reliably persons who exhibit a characteristic Type A behavior pattern. Moreover, it is also clear that such persons are at increased risk of developing clinical manifestations of CHD in comparison to their Type B counterparts. The currently available evidence also suggests that, in addition to clinical events, Type A individuals are more likely than Type Bs to have severe coronary atherosclerosis. Evidence is beginning to accumulate that suggests that Type As are hyperresponsive to behavioral challenges in terms of a wide variety of cardiovascular and neuroendocrine parameters.

During a cholera epidemic in nineteenth-century London, before Pasteur's demonstrations of the germ theory of disease, the noted physician Sir John Snow remarked that all the new cases of cholera were appearing in districts supplied by only one of the three water companies serving the city. When he proposed to close down that water company, he was ridiculed, since the cause of cholera was unknown at the time and most people scoffed at the idea that the drinking water had anything to do with it. Sir John took matters into his own hands and broke the pump handle in one of the neighborhoods supplied by the suspect water company. Within a short time, the rate of new cholera cases in that neighborhood began to show a sharp decline, while the rate in areas that continued to obtain their water from that company remained high. At the present time, we are just about as far along (maybe a bit further!) in our understanding of what it is in Type A behavior that is causing CHD—we know that there is something about Type A behavior that is bad for the heart. It is the task of the next 20 years of research in this area to identify that "something."

Just as the basic science of microbiology eventually was brought to bear in identifying the vibrio comma bacterium as the causative agent in that drinking water, our task is now one of calling upon the various branches of basic behavioral science to help explain what it is in Type A behavior that is pathogenic. There are several promising leads at present: It may be heightened physiological and neuroendocrine responsivity to environmental challenges; it may be an underlying personality characteristic of hostility; more likely, it will prove to be a combination of such characteristics.

In an extensive series of related studies, Glass has brought the principles and techniques of social psychology to bear on this problem (Glass, 1977). He and his colleagues have been able to show that Type A subjects show different behavioral responses compared to Type Bs under conditions of varying task incentives. Using this approach, Blumenthal, McKee, Haney, and Williams (1980) were able to show that the psychomotor performance of Type A and Type B subjects during a verbal problem-solving task did not differ. When a monetary reward was offered, however, the Type A subjects showed significantly greater speed and number of responses in comparison to Type Bs.

PREVENTION, TREATMENT, AND REHABILITATION

Prevention: The Preclinical Phase

With regard to the traditional CHD risk factors—high blood pressure, elevated serum cholesterol, and cigarette smoking—and efforts to reduce their prevalence, it is clear that behavioral factors are of central importance. Major efforts are currently under way in this area, and as it has become evident that simple educational approaches are not sufficiently effective, the input of behavioral scientists has been actively sought. Indeed, a major impetus for the rapid emergence and almost explosive growth of the field of behavioral medicine over the past decade was the realization on the part of leaders in biomedicine (Cooper, Note 1) that proven techniques of behavior modification might be effective in helping people to alter life-styles and behaviors (e.g., reduce saturated fats and cholesterol in the diet, stop smoking, and adhere to antihypertensive regimens) in ways that would reduce risk of CHD. The application of behavioral science knowledge and techniques to the problem of reducing these traditional CHD risk factors represents a major area of behavioral medicine; however, the massive research in these areas and the complexity of the issues involved places any detailed consideration of this area beyond the scope of this volume. Therefore, we shall confine our presentation here to a consideration of only those ways in which behavioral factors are playing a more direct role in issues concerned with prevention, treatment, and rehabilitation. For a detailed consideration of behavioral approaches to the problem of risk factor reduction, the interested reader is referred to several excellent reviews in the areas of compliance with medical regimens (see Haynes, Taylor, & Sackett, 1979), cessation of cigarette smoking (Evans, Hill, Raines, & Henderson, in press), and dietary modification (Stunkard, 1978).

With regard to a direct role for behavioral approaches in the prevention of CHD, the obvious questions are: To what extent can we intervene in the Type A behavior pattern so as to reduce an individual's risk of CHD, and should such intervention be attempted prior to the onset of actual disease (i.e., primary prevention)? Only a few attempts have been made to modify various aspects of the coronary-prone behavior pattern. In 1974, a clinical psychologist, Richard Suinn, published an editorial in the journal *Behavior Therapy* indicating that he had devised a therapeutic program to treat Type A individuals. His approach was basically an anxiety-reduction one, which stressed the fact that Type A persons continually exposed themselves to stress-evoking situations (e.g., deadlines) in order to avoid other even more stressful experiences (e.g., boredom). Thus, he attempted to teach his patients a method of first arousing anxiety in themselves, learning to discriminate the psychological–physiological cues for tension and anxiety, and then learning to reduce the tension state using relaxation skills; he called this program Cardiac Stress Management Training. In addition to training in progressive muscle relaxation, Suinn uses visuomotor (imagery) behavioral rehearsal techniques to teach patients ways of developing and practicing adaptive strategies for handling stressful situations in everyday life. The treatment program is time limited and consists of only five sessions, each an hour long. In his initial study, Suinn (1975) tested the effectiveness of Cardiac Stress Management Training by comparing the relative impact of treatment on both subjective and objective (e.g., changes in lipid levels) indexes of improvement in patients who recently had suffered an MI. He noted that: (*a*) 100% of the treated patients enthusiastically agreed that this type of treatment program should be offered to other cardiac patients, (*b*) 100% of the treated patients felt that they had in fact been helped with tension control, and (*c*) 83% indicated that the training program had helped them change their Type A life-style to a significant degree (Suin , 1974, 1975). Also, there was a notable reduction in blood lipid levels for treated patients, as compared to no-treatment MI patients, such that patients in the treatment group evidenced a 10% reduction in median cholesterol levels compared to a zero change for no-treatment patients and a 27% decrease in triglyceride levels as contrasted with an 11% decrease for no-treatment patients.

In a second study, Suinn and Bloom (1978) demonstrated that cardiac stress management training could be effectively used in alteringType A behavior(s) in persons who had not as yet experienced any CHD but who were at risk by virtue of their Type A profile. These authors studied the effect of stress management training in seven Type A persons, comparing changes in various parameters of coronary-prone behavior and associated physiological findings with those of seven matched no-treatment Type A individuals. The results indicated that (a) treatment led to a significant reduction in hard-driving scores on the JAS, (b) treated patients tended to show a decrease in the speed–impatience factor on the JAS, (c) treatment led to a significant decrease in both situation (state) and trait anxiety, but (d) absolutely no changes were noted as a result of treatment efforts either for systolic or diastolic blood pressure or for blood lipids (cholesterol, triglyceride). On the contrary, there seemed to be a slight increase in the lipid levels for treatment patients.

In a similar study investigating treatment of Type A persons who had not yet experienced clinical CHD, Roskies, Spevack, Surkis, Cohen, and Gilman (1978) compared the effects of both a behavioral and a psychotherapeutic intervention program in a group of 27 professional persons identified by the structured interview as being coronary prone. Their data showed that after 14 sessions of either type of treatment: (a) both groups were equally successful in achieving improved serum cholesterol levels, systolic blood pressure, feelings of time pressure, life satisfaction scores, and tendencies to be preoccupied with somatic concerns, (b) neither treatment approach was able to modify diastolic blood pressure, serum triglycerides, or state–trait anxiety, and (c) most importantly, the therapeutic effects were achieved without modifying factors associated with physical risk for CHD, namely diet, smoking, and exercise.

A wide variety of behavioral techniques have been proposed as potentially useful in reducing Type A behavior (Gentry, 1978). These include *positive reinforcement* (primarily self-reward) for Type B behaviors, such as taking walks in the park or browsing through bookstores and art galleries; *avoidance responding* (taking off one's watch to avoid a sense of time urgency); *response-cost procedures* (self-imposed penalties for behaving in a Type A manner); *thought-stopping techniques* to counteract negative thoughts about competing with others and about having insufficient time to complete multiple activities; a variety of other *relaxation procedures*, including biofeedback and transcendental meditation; and *cognitive behavior modification* aimed either generally at altering one's philosophy about one's relationship to the surrounding environment (Rosenman & Friedman, 1977) or specifically at subcomponents of coronary-prone behavior, such as thoughts about time urgency or thoughts of hostility and competition (Williams *et al.*, 1980).

At Mt. Zion Hospital in San Francisco, Meyer Friedman and others have undertaken a prospective 5-year study (1978–1983) in which 900 Type A men who had recently had an MI were recruited to participate in a program designed to prevent the occurrence of subsequent coronary events. Six hundred men were randomly assigned to an intensive behavior modification program designed to reduce all aspects of the Type A behavior pattern using techniques like those described in the preceding paragraph. The other 300 men were assigned to groups that received conventional education regarding the need to reduce traditional risk factors and group psychotherapy to deal with problems of anxiety and depression. This study is still in progress, and only preliminary results are available thus far. Nevertheless, these preliminary results are quite promising, suggesting rates of reinfarction and death in the Type A behavior modification group that are significantly lower than those for the education–group psychotherapy controls as well as lower than those for a larger sample of controls from the Multiple Risk Factor Intervention Trial (MRFIT) program. Should subsequent analysis of the data from this study confirm the validity of these preliminary findings, the application of the behavioral science techniques utilized in the Mt. Zion study could have a dramatic beneficial impact on morbidity and mortality rates among post-MI patients. With regard to cost–benefit analysis, it is worth noting that the NIH-sponsored Hypertension Detection and Follow-up Program required nearly 11,000 patients and $70 million to demonstrate a beneficial effect of treatment of mild hypertension in terms of reducing subsequent MI. The Mt. Zion project, should the preliminary findings be confirmed, will have required only 900 patients and some $700,000 to demonstrate a beneficial effect of the Type A behavior modification program.

Turning briefly to primary prevention, Blumenthal, Williams, Williams, and Wallace (1980) reported the results of a 10-week program of gradually increasing exercise in a sample of 46 healthy men and women. Over the course of the program, they observed (a) an increase in HDL-cholesterol (felt to be protective against CHD), (b) objective improvement in cardiovascular performance on exercise testing, (c) a significant weight loss, (d) reduction in blood pressure, and (e) a significant reduction in Type A score on the JAS. Interestingly, the significant reduction in JAS Type A score could be accounted for entirely by the Type A subjects in the sample, whose Type A score decreased from a baseline of +9.6 to a level of +6.2 after the 10-week exercise program; in contrast, the Type B subjects score on the Type A scale of the JAS remained stable at −7.2 from before to after the program.

Although all the results reported in this section on modification of the Type A behavior pattern must be considered as preliminary, with final acceptance awaiting validation in extensive further investigation, the results available to date are promising in indicating that systematic application of behavioral techniques can be effective in reducing elements of Type A behavior as well as levels of other indexes of CHD risk.

Treatment: The Clinical Phase

The role of behavioral factors in the clinical phase of CHD can be examined with respect to prehospital behavior and the acute care phase, as well as with regard to the choice of the appropriate treatment modalities to achieve reduction in morbidity and mortality.

Prehospital Behavior

Thousands of persons die suddenly each year as a result of MI and other complications of CHD. It is thought that over 50% of these persons who die do so within 1 hr after the acute symptoms of chest pain, shortness of breath, and fatigue have appeared. Medically, such deaths are associated with ventricular fibrillation occurring during the early phases of infarction, a condition which is potentially treatable and reversible if attended to in time. Psychologically, sudden cardiac deaths appear to be the consequence of faulty decision making on the part of the patient, physician, and family, which is in turn related to a pathological use of denial by persons wishing to avoid the compelling realities of traumatic illness.

Typically, persons experiencing symptoms of CHD (acute MI) delay seeking appropriate medical assistance beyond the crucial 1-hr interval associated with sudden cardiac death (Moss & Goldstein, 1970). That is, the average time period between symptom onset and admission to a medical facility is approximately three hours, ranging from one hour to several days. In one study of CHD patients admitted to a coronary care unit (CCU), at least 50% took longer than 24 hours to seek help (Gentry & Haney, 1975).

Most of the delay in hospital arrival time has been referred to as *decision time,* the interval during which CHD patients: (*a*) must work through a complex cognitive sequence of perception–recognition–realization (Moss, Wynac, & Goldstein, 1969) regarding the nature and severity of their symptoms and the need for treatment, (*b*) engage in self-treatment using a variety of prescribed and patent medications (Simon, Feinleib, & Thompson, 1972), and (*c*) engage in lay communication with spouse, family, and friends to solicit advice on how to cope with the symptoms. This is also the interval when psychological factors play their most important role in affecting patient behavior.

Delay in seeking proper, life-saving assistance is greatest when CHD patients misattribute their "hard" or "soft" symptoms to problems other than the heart and/or when they depend on others in their immediate environment ultimately to make the decision to seek necessary care. Persons who recognize that something is wrong with their heart, upon experiencing severe chest pain, seek help sooner than do persons who displace the cause of their symptoms to diseases of other organ systems (Hackett & Cassem, 1969), for example, gallbladder disease, diabetes, ulcers, common cold, indigestion, and emphysema. The tendency to misidentify the origin of the cardiac symptoms unfortunately characterizes about 70% of patients experiencing either an initial or repeat MI. Denial—that is, the tendency to repudiate or minimize the true meaning of the illness condition—seems to be the primary factor leading to misattribution and thus unnecessary delay. Hackett and Cassem (1969) have shown that patients operating under "minimal denial" more often attribute their symptoms to the heart and generally make the decision to seek help themselves, as opposed to "major deniers," who most frequently list indigestion as the cause of their chest pain and shortness of breath and who also require advice and encouragement from family and friends before seeking medical attention.

Denial interacts with such other factors as death concern, degree of perceived illness, and history of CHD in affecting decision making in patients experiencing symptoms of acute MI (Alonzo, 1973). Patients classified as nondeniers (i.e., they readily and openly admit to being anxious, afraid, and apprehensive during the prehospital phase of illness) and who admit to a high level of death concern almost always make the decision to get medical care themselves; whereas those classified as deniers and as having a low level of death concern rely on the judgment of others. Similarly, patients who are nondeniers and who perceive themselves as seriously ill are generally self-referrals; patients using extreme denial and/or who view themselves as reasonably well despite their symptoms, on the other hand, require advice from others. Finally, 100% of patients described as nondeniers who also have a history of CHD make the decision to seek medical attention themselves, compared with only 25% of those classified as deniers who do not have a positive history of CHD.

The social context in which the patient finds himself and the presence of prodromal symptoms (dizziness, malaise, anorexia) can also interact with denial to foster delay and indecision in the CHD patient. A person first experiencing symptoms of acute MI at work, during a weekday, and in the presence of others is much more likely to delay less. This is presumably because others around him are able to provide corrective feedback concerning the nature and severity of the symptoms and offer advice as to how to respond properly to such symptoms, thereby offsetting the denial that might otherwise determine the patient's course of action. Similarly, patients with a history of angina and other prodromal symptoms tend to take longer to seek help than do those patients without prodromal symptoms, in part because they are able to deny the fact that there is anything seriously wrong with them; that is, they cannot distinguish "the same old symptoms from something new and different," and thus they are prone to inaction.

One way to deal with the problem of denial during the prehospital phase is through education of the patient, his family, and his physician. Patients and their families must learn to recognize the common signs of CHD, those that appear during the prodromal period and in the acute phase; for example, they should know that chest pain is by far the most common symptom of acute MI and they should not be falsely reassured (denial) if the patient has not as yet experienced difficulties in breathing, nausea, extreme weakness and fatigue, and so forth. Whether or not they can distinguish "new symptoms from old," they should be taught to take quick action and not delay or be indecisive about the need for assistance after the onset of symptoms. If the patient cannot accept the reality of his symptoms, for example, if he insists on trying out numerous "home remedies" including various distracting activities and medications, then the family and/or physician (if contacted) should confront the patient with the true nature and severity of his illness and help decide the best, most prompt course of action.

Acute Care Phase

A systematic review of the literature dealing with the psychosocial aspects of recovery from CHD (Doehrman, 1977) has indicated that psychological problems are evident in a reasonably large percentage of persons found in a coronary care unit (CCU) and that they in fact can be associated with outcome variables of morbidity and mortality if not attended to at the time. In some studies only a few CCU patients have shown signs of anxiety (Dominion & Dobson, 1969; Graham, 1969), while in others most if not all of the patients experienced some degree of emotional upset (Hackett, Cassem, & Wishnie, 1968; Cassem & Hackett, 1971). Hackett, Cassem, and Wishnie (1968), for example, found that *at least* 80% of CCU patients demonstrated some signs of being anxious, 58% were depressed, 22% were hostile, and 16% were noticeably agitated. However, these authors further emphasized that the observed level of anxiety was relatively low and that it was unusual for CCU patients to spontaneously complain about being upset. Elsewhere, Cassem and Hackett (1971) have noted that only 33% of CCU patients require psychiatric consultation to resolve their psychological problems.

In fact, most of the emotional problems seen during the acute phase of CHD are short lived and center around a basic concern with death, which is usually resolved after a day or two on the CCU; that is, the patient either lives or dies, and if he lives, his physician reassures him that he is for the most part out of immediate danger. A study by Gentry, Foster, and Haney (1972) found that certain CCU patients were extremely anxious on day 1 after admission to the hospital but that this level of anxiety quickly decreased into a normal range. Similarly, Cassem and Hackett (1971) reported that anxiety is the predominant affect characterizing the CCU patient during the first 2 days in the coronary unit but that it dissipates thereafter, often replaced by a state of depression. Gentry and Haney (1975) subsequently found that the self-reported anxiety found in CCU patients during the first day or so was essentially tied to concerns about death. Patients who reported high levels of death concern also evidenced (*a*) a high level of verbalized subjective anxiety, (*b*) physiological stress (urinary sodium and potassium values), (*c*) more self-reported pain and discomfort, and (*d*) a greater degree of perceived illness.

Interestingly, anxiety not only appears to be the predominant psychological problem associated with the acute phase of CHD but also appears to be unrelated to depression, the second most common emotional disturbance found in this setting (Froese, Hackett, & Cassem, 1974; Gentry *et al.,* 1972). Rather, once CCU patients realize that they have survived their CHD event, they are prone to feelings of depression resulting from increasing thoughts about loss of function experienced during the rehabilitation phase of illness. The depression in most cases has a gradual onset, first appearing in the late stages of the CCU experience (Cassem & Hackett, 1971), increasing when the patient is released to a less intensive cardiology ward (Klein, Kliner, Zipes, Troyer, & Wallace, 1968), and becoming a primary problem after the patient returns home (Cay, Vetter, & Philip, 1970).

To a large extent, anxiety—as well as other emotions found in CCU patients—is related to the patient's use of denial as a defense mechanism. Gentry *et al.* (1972), for example, found that deniers were significantly less anxious across the first 5 days on the CCU than were nondeniers, the latter group of patients reporting a level of anxiety equivalent to that seen in psychiatric patients diagnosed as suffering from anxiety reaction. Denial also affected CCU patients' ratings of perceived health status, again with nondeniers seeing themselves as much sicker on day 1 than did deniers, who reported little change in their health status from the time just prior to their CHD event.

Other factors that determine the presence and severity of emotional disturbance in CCU patients include sociodemographic variables, such as age (Rosen & Bibring, 1966), race/education (Gentry & Haney, 1975) and social class (Rosen & Bibring, 1966; Croog & Levine, 1969); premorbid psychiatric history (Cay, Vetter, & Philip, 1972); medical variables, such as illness severity (Garrity & Klein, 1971; Vetter, Cay, Philip, & Strange, 1977) and prior history of CHD (Gentry & Haney, 1975; Rosen & Bibring, 1966); and situational variables, such as type of CCU environment—open versus closed wards (Leigh, Hofer, Cooper, & Reiser, 1972), witnessing of cardiac arrests in other patients, the experience of cardiac monitoring (Hackett, Cassem, & Wishnie, 1968), and lack of privacy.

Finally, and perhaps most important, there is indication that denial and anxiety have some bearing on morbidity and mortality during the acute phase of

CHD. Gentry *et al.* (1972) observed that two of the eight CCU patients characterized in their initial study as nondeniers died within the first 6 months after
discharge from the hospital; whereas none of the eight patients classified as
deniers died during this same period. Similarly, Hackett *et al.* (1968) reported a
small but significant percentage of deaths in those CCU patients whom they
diagnosed as using "minimal denial." Finally, Cromwell, Butterfield, Brayfield,
and Curry (1977) found that MI patients who displayed extensive scanning
while in the CCU—presumably a reflection of nondenial—were more likely to
suffer a recurrent MI on follow-up.

Choice of Treatment

With regard to treatment of patients who already have clinically evident
CHD, the critical issues are to relieve anginal pain and to reduce mortality. At
present the key treatment choice is between medical management (propranolol,
nitroglycerin, antiarrhythmics) and saphenous vein aorta–coronary bypass
surgery. A number of studies (Hammermeister, DeRouen, & Dodge, 1979;
Harris, Harrell, Lee, Dehar, & Rosati, 1979; Kloster, Kremkau, Ritzmann,
Rahimtoola, Rosch, & Kanarek, 1979; Whalen, Wallace, McNeer, Rosati, &
Lee, 1977) have found that, except for patients with lesions of the left main
coronary artery, prognosis for survival is not different with medical versus
surgical management, especially with control for differential proportions in
each treatment group with impaired left ventricular function. What is clear
from these studies is that surgical treatment is superior to medical treatment
with regard to relief of anginal pain. Thus, except for the small proportion of
patients (approximately 10%) with atherosclerotic involvement of the left main
coronary artery, the main indication for surgical treatment at present is to
achieve relief of anginal pain.

Currently, there are few reliable physiological factors that predict with any
degree of certainty who is likely to achieve significant reduction of angina with
either medical or surgical treatment. Since the phenomenon of pain has long
been known to have a significant psychological–behavioral component, it seems
promising that the application of behavioral science knowledge and techniques
could help to identify subgroups of patients more likely to obtain pain relief
with either of the two currently available forms of treatment. In a study currently under way at Duke, an extensive array of psychosocial and behavioral
variables has been assessed in over 1300 patients referred for diagnostic coronary arteriography. Preliminary analyses of these data suggest that independent
of anatomic and hemodynamic predictors there are psychosocial predictors that
are strongly related to the pain outcome. With medical treatment, patients who
are working at the time they come for their arteriogram are nearly twice as
likely to be pain free at a 6-month follow-up than are patients who are not

working at the time they come for arteriography. Both medically and surgically treated patients who have scores in the normal range on the hysteria scale of the Minnesota Muliphasic Personality Inventory are about equally likely to be pain free at a 6-month follow-up: 85% in the surgically treated group versus 75% of the medically treated patients. Surgically treated patients with scores in the abnormally high range on the hysteria scale show a fall to 70% in the proportion achieving pain relief; this effect is much more pronounced in the medically treated patients with abnormally high hysteria scores who show only 40% achieving pain relief. In view of this relatively greater superiority of surgical over medical management for patients with abnormally high hysteria scores, it is somewhat ironic that patients with hysteria scores in the high range are significantly more likely to be treated medically than surgically. This is probably a function of how these patients with high hysteria scores present—they undoubtedly come across as having an "emotional overlay" upon observation by the cardiologists and surgeons who are charged with making the treatment decisions. It is, perhaps, not surprising that the complaints of such patients are often not taken as seriously as those of patients with fewer hysterical characteristics. The findings cited here suggest, however, that these patients would do far better with surgical than with medical management. In contrast, patients with low hysteria scores might do nearly as well with medical as with surgical management.

It is clear that acceptance of the preliminary findings cited in this section and any detailed consideration of their implications for treatment selection must await their evaluation and publication through the peer review process, as well as their replication in subsequent patients and in other centers. They do suggest, however, the directions and the kinds of impact that we might expect with widespread application of behavioral science approaches to the critical issue of treatment selection in patients with documented coronary disease. With the annual cost of coronary bypass graft surgery currently over $1 billion in the United States, any improvement in our ability to prospectively identify patients who will achieve relief of angina equally as well with medical as with surgical management could result in a dramatic savings in treatment costs.

The Rehabilitation Phase

A large literature is available describing the impact of psychological factors on the CHD patient's course of rehabilitation (Doehrman, 1977; Gulledge, 1975) during the first 12–18 months after discharge from the hospital. Studies have examined the role of such factors as anxiety and depression in impeding the CHD patient's return to normal sexual, work, and recreational functioning and for the most part suggest that psychological factors are only minimally involved in determining to what extent patients resume a healthy and productive life.

Work

The studies describing the course of returning to work after an episode of CHD illustrate this last point quite nicely. A review of the literature in this area (Fisher, 1970; Gordon, 1967; Gulledge, 1975; Hinohara, 1970; Mulcahy, Hickey, & Coghlan, 1972; Nagle, Gangola, & Picton-Robinson, 1971; Sharland, 1964; Weinblatt, Shapiro, Frank, & Sage, 1966; Wenger, Hellerstein, Blackburn, & Castronova, 1973; Wishnie, Hackett, & Cassem, 1971; Wynn, 1967) indicates that most (approximately 80–90%) CHD patients return to work within the first year after their illness. Roughly 50% are back to work at the end of 3 months, 75–80% by 6 months, and 90% at the end of 1 year. A number of variables can interfere with whether or not an individual returns to work, if only to delay his or her return past the point where cardiovascular factors play a role in keeping them at home. These variables include age, severity of cardiac damage, socioeconomic status, level of physical stamina, and psychological status. For purposes of this chapter, we will cover only the impact of psychological factors here.

Fisher (1970) noted that 19% of MI patients in one study failed to return to work but indicated that these patients did not differ from those who did return to work in terms of anxiety level. Wynn (1967), on the other hand, studied some 400 patients with CHD, including hypertensive disease, and found notable emotional distress leading to vocational disability in approximately 50% of them. He suggested that most of these patients (32% of the total sample) were experiencing profound psychological problems, including anxiety and depression, that were interfering with their return to a satisfactory day-to-day pattern of living. Nagle and co-workers (1971) found that 26% of patients failed to return to work at 4 months after an MI and that emotional factors played a primary role in roughly half of these cases (12% of the total sample). Hinohara, (1970) reported that 20% of acute MI patients experiencing their first attack experienced sufficient anxiety to delay their return to work during the first 2 years after their illness. In the majority of cases, anxiety was directly tied to excessive fear of death or recurrence of CHD. Wishnie *et al.* (1971) noted that about 46% of patients followed up after discharge from a CCU failed to return to work as quickly as one might expect but that only 10% of these patients listed anxiety as a major problem (5% of total sample). Gordon (1967) similarly found that depression was only one of many factors accounting for CHD patients' failure to return to work after 1 year, along with age, inability to change jobs, being fired, having other major physical illnesses, and death. Finally, Wenger and colleagues (1973) reported that only 13% of patients with uncomplicated MI failed to return to work at the end of 1 year and that only about 25% of these patients (3.5% of total sample) failed to do so because of profound psychological disturbance. In short, these findings suggest that, at most, psychological factors can account for between 3% and 12% of the persons who fail to return to normal, satisfying work relationships within the first year post-MI. This is, of course, with the one notable exception of the Wynn (1967) study, which can in part be explained by the fact that the patients in this sample were screened from lower socioeconomic classes (semiskilled and unskilled workers) and were referred in part because they were having difficulty in returning to work.

Sexual Activity

As was true of return to work after CHD, the literature describing return to sexual activity is for the most part encouraging and indicates that psychological factors do not play a major role in affecting outcome in this area of rehabilitation (Fisher, 1970; Hellerstein & Friedman, 1970; Massie, 1969; Scalzi, Loya, & Golden, 1977; Stern, Note 2). Hellerstein and Friedman (1970), for example, have shown that the level of sexual activity seen in persons within the first year after an MI is about 80% of what it was before illness (i.e., number of orgasms per week). Virtually all the patients in their classic study reported some level of sexual function 1 year after discharge from the hospital; 42% returned to the same level of intercourse, while the remaining 58% showed some decline in such activity. Interestingly, 25% of these patients showed an improvement in the quality of sexual performance as a result of their CHD episode. Hellerstein and Friedman noted that patients decreasing their sexual activity indicated a variety of reasons for this: loss of sexual interest or desire (39%), spouse's reluctance to cooperate (25%), depression (21%), anxiety about recurrence of CHD (18%) and/or coital death, and anxiety resulting from cardiovascular symptoms (angina, tachycardia) commonly associated with sexual activity post-MI.

In another study, Stern (Note 2) showed that some 69% of MI patients returned to normal sexual activity during the first year after infarction, but with striking differences between depressed and nondepressed individuals. That is, 93% of the nondepressed patients were able to successfully resume sexual activity without difficulty during this first year, but only 58% of the depressed patients were able to resume some level of sexual intercourse during this same time period. Stern further emphasized the role of denial as a defense mechanism against depressive affect in these patients, linking it to a more positive rehabilitation status in much the same way other studies have linked it to successful adaptation in the intensive, acute care phase of illness (Gentry *et al.*, 1972).

Depression is a significant psychological factor affecting return to sexual function because it directly contributes to a decline in sexual interest and because it can have diminished libido as a symptom. Extreme fatigue, another sign of depression, may also be seen by some CHD patients as a reason for not resuming sexual activity quickly or to the same degree as prior to their illness.

Recreation

Even though return to social–recreational activities is a vital part of cardiac rehabilitation, little if any information is currently available describing the impact of psychological factors on such activities in the recovering CHD patient. Presumably, if the patient is suffering from depression or undue anxiety about death and recurrent heart problems—problems sometimes associated with a failure to return to work and sexual function—he or she will most certainly also fail to resume normal recreational–social relationships. A loss of interest in sports, extreme feelings of fatigue and weakness, and a drastic change in self-image (e.g., less of a man or woman, less powerful, less athletic)—all signs of depression in a CHD patient—may appear for some indeterminant time after acute MI or other types of CHD.

One study (Rose, 1974) has noted a pathological relationship between certain types of spectator sports and CHD. In this study, 11 postcoronary patients were monitored for irregular cardiovascular activity during their attendance at a football game; 2 of these patients had previously suffered a cardiac arrest in the football stadium and had been resuscitated. Five of the patients (45%) evidenced abnormalities of heart rate, rhythm, and/or ischemic patterns indicating a detrimental effect of such viewing on cardiac function. The remaining 6 patients showed no signs of irregular heart function resulting from this type of recreational activity. Presumably, certain types of personalitiies—emotionally labile, aggressive, competitive—cannot watch such sports without experiencing emotional upset of such a magnitude as to produce coronary dysfunction, placing them at risk for further CHD events.

Similarly, one might speculate that Type A individuals who respond to a coronary event by increasing (rather than reducing) their level of competitive social–recreational activity will be at increased risk for additional coronary disease.

Role of Psychotherapy in Rehabilitation

Few studies have yet been published that assess the effectiveness of psychotherapy, either group or individual, in helping to rehabilitate the CHD patient after an episode of illness (Adsett & Bruhn, 1968; Bilodeau & Hackett, 1971; Ibrahim, Feldman, Sultz, Staiman, Young, & Dean, 1974; Mone, 1970;

Ohlmeier, Karstens, & Kohle, 1973; Rahe, Rufflic, Suchor, & Arthur, 1973). With the exception of a study by Ibrahim and co-workers (1974), most of the studies reporting on the benefits of group psychotherapy for CHD patients have employed only a few sessions (ranging from 6 to 12) of treatment, have lacked any type of no-treatment control group for purposes of comparison, and have failed to fully assess the impact of such treatment on the full range of functions in this particular patient group. For example, one study (Mone, 1970) noted that 10 sessions of group therapy led to a decrease in depression and hypochondriasis (i.e., excessive preoccupation with somatic concerns) in post-MI patients. Another study (Rahe et al., 1973) similarly reported short-term improvement in patients' compliance with the medical regimen, a decrease in smoking, more effective use of nitroglycerine, a decrease in reported angina, and less rehospitalization resulting from therapy after only 6 sessions. Other studies (Adsett & Bruhn, 1968; Bilodeau & Hackett, 1971), however, fail to describe exactly what the benefits of such treatment are for these patients.

In the Ibrahim and co-workers (1974) study, a total of 118 patients were randomly assigned to five different therapy groups and a no-treatment control group, which met on a weekly basis for a period of 18 months post-MI. The patients for the most part attended the groups faithfully (70% average attendance), and there were few persons who refused to participate (16% of those invited) and also few dropouts (15% of those who began). The results of the study suggested that less social alienation was experienced by patients in the therapy groups than by control patients during this period. In addition, there appeared to be a general decline in levels of competition and exaggerated feelings of responsibility (e.g., as seen in Type As) for those patients receiving therapy. However, these effects were short lived in that most therapy patients had returned to their previous levels of stressful behavior 6 months after the termination of treatment. Apparently what had been learned in treatment could not be retained once the patient was on his or her own without the support of others in a similar situation.

Ibrahim (1976) elsewhere notes that group therapy for CHD patients generally involves discussion of five main issues: fear of death, physical condition (cardiac status), work, domestic relationships, and personal life-style preferences (e.g., dealing with diet, exercise, smoking, and sexual activity). He also points out an important issue, that is,

> the term "group therapy" is a misnomer. In these sessions, the therapist serves as a catalyst fostering free interaction and encouraging the expression of emotions. Education, support, reinforcement, learning from and helping one another, free expression of anger, etc., are the substance of discussion during the sessions [p. 25].

This is the same point made by Gruen (1975) in his description of individual psychotherapy with CHD patients in the CCU. He suggests that effective therapy in this setting should focus on, among other things, (a) the development of a genuine interest in the CHD patient and an understanding of his positive qualities—those that will lead to successful coping and adaptation to the illness condition, and (b) a mixture of reassurance, reflection, reinforcement, and encouragement for attempts by the patient to master his own conflicts and dilemmas generated by the cardiac episode.

Rather than using one of the various forms of psychotherapy, applied with the general goal of reducing anxiety and depression among post-MI patients, the study of Friedman and co-workers described earlier, in the section on prevention, utilizes behavior modification techniques specifically directed toward reduction of all aspects of Type A behavior. As noted, the preliminary findings of this intervention study suggest that the behavior modification approach is more effective in reducing mortality than is a more traditional group psychotherapy approach.

CONCLUSIONS

The evidence supporting the role of behavioral factors in all stages of disease—etiology and pathogenesis, the clinical phase, and the rehabilitation phase—is stronger for CHD than for any other physical disorder. Type A behavior is now officially sanctioned as a risk factor for CHD, and intensive research efforts are under way to identify the pathogenic mechanisms underlying this relationship. Behavior modification techniques appear to offer the best promise for reduction of life-styles and behaviors that have been found to be risk factors for CHD. Behavioral and psychological assessment has much to offer with regard to identification of prognostically homogeneous subgroups of CHD patients. Realization of this potential could lead to more effective selection of patients for various treatment modalities—behavioral as well as surgical and pharmacologic. Not only are behavioral factors playing a role in the outcome of the rehabilitation phase of CHD, behavioral intervention techniques are also showing promise of becoming important active ingredients of the comprehensive approach to the post-MI patient.

Clearly, behavioral medicine has much to offer for the reduction of morbidity and mortality associated with CHD, the nation's number one public health problem.

REFERENCE NOTES

1. Cooper, T. Coming national policy on prevention of heart diseases. Paper presented to Medical Dietetic Symposium, University of Arizona, March 1973.

2. Stern, M. J. *Psychosocial responses of patients: Post-myocardial infarction.* Paper presented at the annual meeting of the American Psychosomatic Society, Philadelphia, April 1974.
3. Williams, R. B., Lane, J. D., White, A. D., Kuhn, C. M., & Schanberg, S. M. *Type A behavior pattern and neuroendocrine response during mental work.* Paper presented at the annual meeting of the American Psychosomatic Society, Boston, March 1981.

REFERENCES

Adsett, C. A., & Bruhn, J. G. Short-term group psychotherapy for myocardial patients and their wives. *Canadian Medical Association Journal,* 1968, *99,* 577.
Alonzo, A. A. *Illness behavior during acute episodes of coronary heart disease.* Unpublished PhD dissertation, University of California, Berkeley, 1973.
Arlow, J. A. Identification mechanisms in coronary occlusions. *Psychosomatic Medicine,* 1945, *7,* 195–209.
Berkman, L. F., & Syme, S. L. Social networks, host resistance and mortality: A nine-year follow-up study of Alameda County residents. *American Journal of Epidemiology,* 1979, *109,* 186–204.
Bilodeau, C. B., & Hackett, T. P. Issues raised in a group setting by patients recovering from myocardial infarction. *American Journal of Psychiatry,* 1971, *128,* 105.
Blumenthal, J. A., McKee, D. C., Haney, T., & Williams, R. B. Task incentives, type A behavior pattern, and verbal problem solving performance. *Journal of Applied Social Psychology,* 1980, *10,* 101–114.
Blumenthal, J. A., Williams, R. B., Kong, Y., Schanberg, S. M., & Thompson, L. W. Type A behavior and angiographically documented coronary disease. *Circulation,* 1978, *58,* 634–639.
Blumenthal, J. A., Williams, R. S., Williams, R. B., & Wallace, A. G. The effects of exercise on the Type A behavior pattern. *Psychosomatic Medicine,* 1980, *42,* 289–296.
Brand, R. J. Coronary prone behavior as an independent risk factor for coronary heart disease. In T. M. Dembroski, S. M. Weiss, J. L. Shields, S. C. Haynes, M. Feinleib. *Coronary-prone behavior.* New York: Springer-Verlag, 1978.
Cassem, N. H., & Hackett, T. P. Psychiatric consultation in a coronary care unit. *Annals of Internal Medicine,* 1971, *75,* 9–39.
Cay, E. L., Vetter, N. J., & Philip, A. E. Psychological reactions to a coronary care unit. *Scandinavian Journal of Rehabilitation Medicine,* 1970, *23,* 78–86.
Cay, E. L., Vetter, N. J., & Philip, A. E. Psychological status during recovery from an acute care unit. *Journal of Psychosomatic Research,* 1972, *16,* 425.
Cobb, S. Social support as a moderator of life stress. *Psychosomatic Medicine,* 1976, *38,* 300–314.
Cook, W. W., & Medley, D. M. Proposed hostility and pharisaic-virtue scales for the MMPI. *Journal of Applied Psychology,* 1954, *38,* 414–418.
Cromwell, R. L., Butterfield, E. C., Brayfield, T. M., & Curry, J. J. *Acute myocardial infarction— Reaction and recovery.* St. Louis: Mosby, 1977.
Croog, S. H., & Levine, S. Social status and subjective perceptions of 250 men after myocardial infarction. *Public Health Reports* 1969, *84,* 989.
Dembroski, T. M., MacDougall, J. M., Herd, J. A., & Shields, J. L. Effect of level of challenge on pressor and heart rate responses in Type A and B subjects. *Journal of Applied Social Psychology,* 1978, *9,* 209–228.
Dembroski, T. M., MacDougall, J. M., Shields, J. L., Petitto, J., & Lushene, R. Components of the Type A coronary-prone behavior pattern and cardiovascular responses to psychomotor performance challenge. *Journal of Behavioral Medicine,* 1978, *1,* 159–175.

Dembroski, T. M., Weiss, S. M., Shields, J. L., Haynes, S. G., & Feinleib, M. *Coronary-prone behavior*. New York: Springer-Verlag, 1978.

Dimsdale, J. E., Hackett, T. P., Hutter, A. M., Block, P. C., & Catanzano, D. Type A personality and extent of coronary atherosclerosis. *American Journal of Cardiology*, 1978, *42*, 583–586.

Doehrman, S. R. Psycho-social aspects of recovery from coronary heart disease: A Review. *Social Science & Medicine*, 1977, *11*, 199–218.

Dohrenwend, B. S., & Dohrenwend, B. P. *Stressful life events: Their nature and effects*. New York: Wiley (Interscience), 1974.

Dunbar, F. *Psychosomatic diagnosis*. New York: Hoeber & Harper, 1943.

Engel, G. Sudden and rapid death during psychological stress. *Annals of Internal Medicine*, 1971, *74*, 771.

Evans, R. I., Hill, P. C., Raines, B. E., & Henderson, A. H. Current psychological, social and educational programs in control and prevention of smoking: A critical methodological review. *Atherosclerosis Review*, in press.

Fisher, I. Impact of physical disability on vocational activity: Work status following myocardial infarction. *Scandinavian Journal of Rehabilitation Medicine*, 1970, *65*, 2–3.

Frank, K. A., Heller, S. S., Kornfeld, D. S., Sporn, A. A., & Weiss, M. B. Type A behavior pattern and coronary angiographic findings. *Journal of American Medical Association*, 1978, *240*, 761–763.

Friedman, M. *The pathogenesis of coronary artery disease*. New York: McGraw-Hill, 1969.

Friedman, M., Byers, S. O., Diament, J., & Rosenman, R. H. Plasma catecholamine response of coronary prone subjects (Type A) to a specific challenge. *Metabolism*, 1975, *24*, 205–210.

Friedman, M., Byers, S. O., & Rosenman, R. H. Plasma ACTH and cortisol concentration of coronary prone subjects. *Proceedings of the Society of Experimental Biology & Medicine*, 1972, *140*, 681–684.

Friedman, M., Byers, S. O., Rosenman, R. H., & Elevitch, F. R. Coronary prone individuals (Type A behavior pattern). Some biochemical characteristics. *Journal of American Medical Association*, 1970, *212*, 1030–1037.

Friedman, M., Byers, S. O., Rosenman, R. H., & Newman, R. Coronary prone individuals (Type A behavior pattern). Growth hormone responses. *Journal of American Medical Association*, 1971, *217*, 929–932.

Friedman, M., & Rosenman, R. H. Association of specific overt behavior pattern with blood and cardiovascular findings. *Journal of American Medical Association*, 1959, *169*, 1286–1296.

Friedman, M., Rosenman, R. H., Straus, R., Wurm, M., & Kositchek, R. The relationship of behavior pattern A to the state of the coronary vasculature: A study of fifty-one autopsy subjects. *American Journal of Medicine*, 1968, *44*, 525–537.

Friedman, M., St. George, S., & Byers, S. O. Excretion of catecholamines, 17-ketosteroids, 17-hydroxy corticoids and 6-hydroxy-indole in men exhibiting a particular behavior pattern (A) associated with high incidence of clinical coronary artery disease. *Journal of Clinical Investigation*, 1960, *39*, 758–764.

Froese, A., Hackett, T. P., & Cassem, N. H. Trajectories of anxiety and depression in denying and nondenying acute myocardial infarction patients during hospitalization. *Journal of Psychosomatic Research*, 1974, *18*, 413.

Garrity, T. F., & Klein, R. F. A behavioral prediction of survival among heart attack patients. In E. Palmore & F. C. Jeffers (Eds.), *Predictions of life-span*. Lexington, Mass: D. C. Heath, 1971.

Gentry, W. D. Behavior modification of coronary-prone behavior pattern. In T. M. Dembroski, S. M. Weiss, J. L. Shields, S. G. Haynes, & M. Feinleib, (Eds.), *Coronary-prone behavior*. New York: Springer-Verlag, 1978.

Gentry, W. D., Foster, S., & Haney, T. Denial as a determinant of anxiety and preceived health status in the coronary care unit. *Psychosomatic Medicine*, 1972, *34*, 39–46.

Gentry, W. D., & Haney, T. L. Emotional and behavioral reaction to acute myocardial infarction. *Heart & Lung,* 1975, *4,* 738–745.

Glass, D. C. *Behavior patterns, stress and coronary disease.* Hillsdale, N.J.: Erlbaum, 1977.

Gordon, B. M. Return to work after myocardial infarction. *Scottish Medical Journal,* 1967, *12,* 297.

Gruen, W. Effects of brief psychotherapy during the hospitalization period on the recovery period in heart attacks. *Journal of Consulting & Clinical Psychology,* 1975, *43,* 223.

Gulledge, A. D. The psychological aftermath of a myocardial infarction. In W. D. Gentry & R. B. Williams (Eds.), *Psychological aspects of myocardial infarction and coronary care.* St. Louis: Mosby, 1975.

Hackett, T. P., & Cassem, N. H. Factors contributing to delay in responding to the signs and symptoms of acute myocardial infarction. *American Journal of Cardiology,* 1969, *24,* 651–659.

Hackett, T. P., Cassem, N. H., & Wishnie, H. A. The coronary care unit. An appraisal of its psychologic hazards. *New England Journal of Medicine,* 1968, *279,* 1365–1369.

Hammermeister, K. E., DeRouen, T. A., & Dodge, H. T. Variables predictive of survival in patients with coronary disease. *Circulation,* 1979, *59,* 421–430.

Harris, P. J., Harrell, F. E., Lee, K. L., Dehar, V. S., & Rosati, R. A. Survival in medically treated coronary artery disease. *Circulation,* 1979, *60,* 1259–1269.

Haynes, R. B., Taylor, O. W., & Sackett, D. L. *Compliance in health care.* Baltimore: Johns Hopkins Press, 1979.

Hellerstein, H. K., & Friedman, E. H. Sexual activity and the postcoronary patient. *Archives of Internal Medicine,* 1970, *125,* 987.

Hinohara, S. Psychological aspects in rehabilitation of coronary heart disease. *Scandinavian Journal of Rehabilitation Medicine,* 1970, *2,* 53.

Ibrahim, M. A. The impact of intervention upon psychosocial functions of post-myocardial infarction patients. *Journal of South Carolina Medical Association,* 1976 (Supplement).

Ibrahim, M. A., Feldman, J. G., Sultz, H. A., Staiman, M. G., Young, L. J., & Dean, D. Management after myocardial infarction. A controlled trial of the effect of group psychotherapy. *International Journal of Psychiatric Medicine,* 1974, *5,* 253.

Jenkins, C. D. Psychologic and social precursors of coronary disease. *New England Journal of Medicine,* 1971, *284,* 244–255, 307–317.

Jenkins, C. D. Recent evidence supporting psychologic and social risk factors for coronary heart disease. *New England Journal of Medicine,* 1976, *249,* 987–994, 1033–1038.

Jenkins, C. D. A comparative review of the interview and questionnaire methods in the assessment of the coronary prone behavior pattern. In T. M. Dembroski, S. M. Weiss, J. L. Shields, S. G. Haynes, & M. Feinleib (Eds.), *Coronary-prone behavior.* New York: Springer-Verlag, 1978.

Jenkins, C. D., Rosenman, R. H., & Friedman, M. Development of an objective psychological test for the determination of the coronary prone behavior pattern in employed men. *Journal of Chronic Disease,* 1967, *20,* 371–379.

Jenkins, C. D., Rosenman, R. H., & Zyzanski, S. J. Prediction of clinical coronary heart disease by a test for the coronary prone behavior pattern. *New England Journal of Medicine,* 1974, *290,* 1271–1275.

Kaplan, B. H., Cassel, J. C., Tyroler, J. A., Cornoni, J. C., Kleinbaum, D. G., & Hames, C. G. Occupational mobility and coronary heart disease. *Archives of Internal Medicine* (Chicago), 1971, *128,* 938–942.

Kannel, W. B., McGee, D., & Gordon, T. A general cardiovascular risk profile: The Framingham Study. *American Journal of Cardiology,* 1976, *38,* 46–51.

Kemple, C. Rorschach method and psychosomatic diagnosis. *Psychosomatic Medicine,* 1945, *7,* 85–89.

Keys, A. The individual risk of coronary heart disease. *Annals of New York Academy of Science,* 1966, *134,* 1046–1063.

Klein, R. F., Kliner, V. A., Zipes, D. P., Troyer, W. G., Jr., & Wallace, A. G. Transfer from a coronary-care unit: Some adverse responses. *Archives of Internal Medicine*, 1968, *122*, 104–110.

Kloster, F. E., Krenkan, E. L., Ritzmann, L. W., Rohimtoola, S. H., Rosch, J., & Kanarek, P. H. Coronary bypass for stable angina. *New England Journal of Medicine*, 1979, *300*, 149–157.

Leigh, H., Hofer, M. A., Cooper, J., & Reiser, M. F. A psychological comparison of patients in "open" and "closed" coronary care units. *Journal of Psychosomatic Research*, 1972, *16*, 449–456.

Manuck, S. B., Craft, R., & Gold, K. Coronary prone behavior pattern and cardiovascular response. *Psychophysiology*, 1978, *15*, 403–411.

Marmot, M. G., & Syme, S. L. Acculturation and coronary heart disease in Japanese-Americans. *American Journal of Epidemiology*, 1976, *104*, 225–247.

Massie, E. Sudden death during coitus—fact or fiction? *Medical Aspects of Human Sexuality*, 1969, *3*, 22.

Matthews, K. A., Glass, D. C., Rosenman, R. H., & Bortner, R. W. Competitive drive, pattern A, and coronary heart disease. A further analysis of some data from the Western Collaborative Group Study. *Journal of Chronic Disease*, 1977, *30*, 489–498.

Medalie, J. H., Kahn, H. A., Neufeld, H. N., Riss, E., Goldbourt, U., Perlstein, T., & Oron, D. Myocardial infarction over a five-year period. I. Prevalence, incidence and mortality experience. *Journal of Chronic Disease*, 1973, *26*, 63–84.

Menninger, K. A., & Menninger, W. C. Psychoanalytic observations in cardiac disorders. *American Heart Journal*, 1936, *11*, 10–21.

Mone, L. Short-term group psychotherapy in post-cardiac patients. *International Journal of Group Psychotherapy*, 1970, *20*, 99.

Moss, A. J., & Goldstein, S. The pre-hospital phase of actue myocardial infarction. *Circulation*, 1970, *41*, 737.

Moss, A. J., Wynar, B., & Goldstein, S. Delay in hospitalization during the acute coronary period. *American Journal of Cardiology*, 1969, *24*, 659–664.

Mulcahy, R., Hickey, N., & Coghlan, N. Rehabilitation of patients with coronary heart disease. *Geriatrics*, 1972, *3*, 120.

Nagle, R., Gangola, R., & Picton-Robinson, I. Factors influencing return to work after myocardial infarction. *Lancet*, 1971, *2*, 454.

NHLBI Forum on Coronary Prone Behavior and Coronary Heart Disease. A critical review. *Report of the coronary prone behavior review panel*. National Heart, Lung and Blood Institute, National Institutes of Health, Washington, D.C., December 1978.

Ohlmeier, D., Karstens, R., & Kohle, K. Psycho-analytic group interview and short-term psychotherapy with postmyocardial infarction patients. *Psychiatric Clinic*, 1973, *6*, 240.

Osler, W. *Lectures on angina pectoris and allied states*. New York: Appleton, 1897.

Osler, W. The Lumlein Lectures on angina pectoris. *Lancet*, 1910, *1*, 839–844.

Rahe, R. Subjects' recent life changes and their near-future illness reports: A review. *Annals of Clinical Research*, 1972, *4*, 250–265.

Rahe, R. H., Rufflic, C. F., Suchor, R. J., & Arthur, R. J. Group therapy in the outpatient management of post-myocardial infarction patients. *International Journal of Psychiatric Medicine*, 1973, *4*, 77.

Rose, K. D. The post-coronary patient as a spectator sportsman. In R. S. Eliot (Ed.), *Stress and heart*. New York: Futura, 1974.

Rosen, J. L., & Bibring, G. L. Psychological reactions to hospitalized male patients to a heart attack. *Psychosomatic Medicine*, 1966, *28*, 808–813.

Rosenman, R. H., Brand, R. J., Jenkins, C. D., Friedman, M., Straus, R., & Wurm, M. Coronary heart disease in the Western Collaborative Group Study: Final follow-up experience of 8 ½ years. *Journal of American Medical Association*, 1975, *233*, 872–877.

Rosenman, R. H., & Friedman, M. Association of specific behavior pattern in women with blood and cardiovascular findings. *Circulation*, 1961, *24*, 1173–1184.

Rosenman, R. H., & Friedman, M. Modifying Type A behavior pattern. *Journal of Psychosomatic Research*, 1977, *21*, 323–331.

Rosenman, R. H., Friedman, M., Straus, R., Wurm, M., Kositchek, R., Hahn, W., & Werthessen, N. T. A predictive study of coronary heart disease. *Journal of American Medical Association*, 1964, *189*, 15–22.

Roskies, E., Spevack, M., Surkis, A., Cohen, C., & Gilman, S. Changing the coronary-prone (Type A) behavior pattern in a nonclinical population. *Journal of Behavioral Medicine*, 1978, 1, 201–216.

Ross, R., & Glomset, J. A. The pathogenesis of atherosclerosis. *New England Journal of Medicine*, 1976, *295*, 369–420.

Scalzi, C. C., Loya, F., & Golden, J. S. Sexual therapy of patients with cardiovascular disease. *Western Journal of Medicine*, 1977, *126*, 237.

Scherwitz, L., Berton, K., & Leventhal, H. Type A behavior, self-involvement, and cardiovascular response. *Psychosomatic Medicine*, 1978, *40*, 593–609.

Sharland, D. C. Ability of men to return to work after cardiac infarction. *British Medical Journal*, 1964, *2*, 718.

Shekelle, R. B., Ostfeld, A. M., & Paul, O. Social status and incidence of coronary heart disease. *Journal of Chronic Disease*, 1969, *22*, 281–294.

Simon, A. B., Feinleib, M., & Thompson, H. R. Components of delay in the pre-hospital phase of acute myocardial infarction. *American Journal of Cardiology*, 1972, *30*, 476–483.

Stunkard, A. J. Symposium on obesity: Basic mechanism and treatment. *Psychiatric Clinics of North America*, 1978, *1*, 1–273.

Spain, D., Brodess, V., & Mohr, C. Coronary atherosclerosis as a cause of unexpected and unexplained death. An autopsy study from 1949–1959. *Journal of American Medical Association*, 1960, *174*, 384.

Suinn, R. M. Behavior therapy for cardiac patients. *Behavior Therapy*, 1974, *5*, 569.

Suinn, R. M. The cardiac stress management program for Type A patients. *Cardiac Rehabilitation*, 1975, *5*, 13–15.

Suinn, R. M., & Bloom, L. J. Anxiety management training for pattern A behavior. *Journal of Behavioral Medicine*, 1978, *1*, 25–36.

Syme, S. L., Borhani, N. O., & Buechley, R. W. Cultural mobility and coronary heart disease in an urban area. *American Journal of Epidemiology*, 1965, *82*, 334–346.

Syme, S. L., Hyman, M. M., & Enterline, P. E. Some social and cultural factors associated with the occurrence of coronary heart disease. *Journal of Chronic Disease*, 1964, *17*, 277–289.

Timberline Conference on Psychophysiologic Aspects of Cardiovascular Disease. *Psychosomatic Medicine*, 1964, *26*, 405–541.

Tyroler, J. A., & Cassel, J. Health consequences of culture change. II. Effect of urbanization on coronary heart mortality in rural residents. *Journal of Chronic Disease*, 1964, *17*, 167–177.

U.S. Department of Health, Education and Welfare. The report by the National Heart and Lung Institute Task Force on Arteriosclerosis, December 1977.

Vetter, N. J., Cay, E. L., Philip, A. E., & Strange, R. C. Anxiety on admission to a coronary care unit. *Journal of Psychosomatic Research*, 1977, *21*, 73–80.

Von Dusch, T. Lehrbuck der Herzksankheiten. Leipzig: Verlag Von Wilhem Engelman, 1868.

Weinblatt, E., Shapiro, S., Frank, C. W., & Sager, R. V. Return to work and work status following first myocardial infarct. *American Journal of Public Health*, 1966, *56*, 169.

Wenger, N. K., Hellerstein, H. K., Blackburn, H., & Castronova, S. J. Uncomplicated myocardial infarct. *Journal of American Medical Association*, 1973, *224*, 511.

Whalen, R. E., Wallace, A. G. McNeer, J. F., Rosati, R. A., & Lee, K. L. The natural history of coronary heart disease: An update on surgical and medical management. *Transactions of the American Clinical and Climatological Association, 1977, 89,* 19–35.

Williams, R. B. Physiologic mechanisms underlying the association between psychosocial factors and coronary heart disease. In W. D. Gentry & R. B. Williams (Eds.), *Psychosocial aspects of myocardial infarction and coronary care.* St. Louis: Mosby, 1975.

Williams, R. B., Friedman, M., Glass, D., Herd, J. A., & Schneiderman, N. Mechanisms linking behavioral and pathophysiological process. In T. M. Dembroski, S. M. Weiss, J. L. Shields, S. G. Haynes, & M. Feinleib (Eds.), *Coronary-prone behavior.* New York: Springer-Verlag, 1978.

Williams, R. B., Haney, T. L., Lee, K. L., Kong, Y., Blumenthal, J. A., & Whalen, R. E. Type A behavior hostility and coronary atherosclerosis. *Psychomatic Medicine, 1980, 42,* 539–549.

Wishnie, H. A., Hackett, T. P., & Cassem, N. H. Psychological hazards of convalescence following myocardial infarction. *Journal of American Medical Association, 1971, 215,* 1292–1297.

Wolfe, S. Psychosocial forces in myocardial infarction and sudden death. In S. Bondurat (Ed.), *Research on acute myocardial infarction.* New York: American Heart Association, 1969.

Wynn, A. Unwarranted emotional distress in men with ischemic heart disease. *Medical Journal of Australia, 1967, 2,* 347.

Zyzanski, S. J., Jenkins, C. D., Ryan, T. J., Flessas, A., & Everist, M. Psychological correlates of coronary angiographic findings. *Archives of Internal Medicine, 1976, 136,* 1234–1237.

6

Hypertension

Hypertension is a major public health problem in the United States, estimated to occur in 10–15% of the general population (Hypertension Detection and Follow-up Program Cooperative Group, 1979). High levels of arterial blood pressure increase the risk of target-organ damage and life-threatening disorders of the heart, kidneys, and blood vessels (Kannel, Gordon, & Schwartz, 1971). A vast proportion of all cases of hypertension are diagnosed as *essential hypertension,* defined by high blood pressure that is not secondary to kidney, endocrine, or other physical disorders. Investigators do not entirely agree about the significance of psychological factors in hypertension, although the disorder is clearly associated with various behavioral, social, and environmental factors (Gutmann & Benson, 1971). The evidence suggests that such factors may play a critical triggering role, particularly for those individuals who show excessive reactivity of the sympathetic nervous system. This reactivity is thought to be associated with elevations of blood pressure in the early stages of hypertension, accompanied by increases in heart rate, cardiac output, and cardiac contractility (Frohlich, Tarazi, & Dustan, 1969; Frohlich, Ulrych, Tarazi, Dustan, & Page, 1967; Julius & Conway, 1968). The excessive reactivity is probably genetic or constitutional in nature. Other evidence indicates important interactions between the autonomic and renin–angiotensin systems that play a significant role in the disorder (Bunag, Page, & McCubbin, 1966; Davis, 1971; Stokes, Goldsmith, Starr, Gentle, Mani, & Stewart, 1970; Ueda, Kaneko, Takeda, Ikeda, & Yagi, 1970; Ueda, Yasuda, Takabatake, Lizuka, Lizuka, Ihori, & Sakamoto, 1970).

Current medical practice dictates drug treatment for elevated blood pressure, especially if there is reason to suspect that the hypertension will become severe and fixed (Freis, 1974; Merrill, 1966; VA Cooperative Study Group on Antihypertensive Agents, 1967, 1970, 1972). Long-term research completed in

129

the late 1970s suggests that active drug treatment of mild hypertension (90–105 mm Hg diastolic) can significantly reduce mortality rate, stroke, heart disease, and other complications (Hypertension Detection and Follow-up Program Cooperative Group, 1979).

In view of the environmental, behavioral, and autonomic nervous system components of hypertension, behavioral approaches offer a nonpharmacologic means of lowering pressure. Two important problems in the management of hypertension, besides detection and diagnosis, are effectiveness of drug therapy and treatment compliance. Behavioral treatments are important in cases where drug control is not adequate or results in disturbing side effects. Such treatments may be added to drug treatment to provide greater control of blood pressure and to reduce required drug dosage. Or behavioral treatments may be of particular value for patients who do not want to comply with drug treatment for whatever reasons. Thus, behavioral techniques may increase the number of treated patients, aid in prevention, and generally help make patients more aware of responsibility for their health.

PATHOPHYSIOLOGY OF HYPERTENSION

A discussion of interacting systems and processes involved in the regulation of systemic arterial pressure is given in Chapter 4 (see Figure 4.3). In normal states, the cardiovascular system serves to maintain homeostasis; its principal physiological function is to provide adequate cell nutrients to the body tissues in response to metabolic demands. The cardiovascular system is finely regulated to maintain cell nutrients proportional to tissue metabolic requirements by means of control of cardiac output, systemic arterial pressure usually remaining within narrow limits. Blood pressure changes when metabolic demands are excessive, such as during exercise. The metabolic-dependent regulation of the cardiovascular system is easily overriden by cortical or subcortical stimulation under "stress" conditions or in preparation for exercise or "action" (Brod, 1964; Folkow & Rubinstein, 1966). Systemic arterial blood pressure is significantly influenced by stress and other environmental demands (as discussed later). Such neurogenic influences, perfectly adaptive where action follows the preparatory rise in cardiovascular activity, are not adaptive in typical life situations where fight or flight responses are not compatible with accepted social behavior. Neurogenic factors have often been postulated as being implicated in the hypertensive process (DeQuattro & Miura, 1973; Dustan, Tarazi, & Bravo, 1972; Esler, Julius, Zweifler, Randall, Harburg, Gardiner, & DeQuattro, 1977; Pfeffer & Frohlich, 1973).

In essential hypertension, blood pressure is elevated above certain arbitrary age–sex norms. The pressure tends to increase ("hypertension begets hypertension"), and the whole system stabilizes again and again around higher and higher levels of blood pressure (Rushmer, 1970). In a normal organism, the system compensates to reduce acute increases in blood pressure or cardiac output to normal levels.

The complexity of physiological factors thought to be involved in the development or maintenance of essential hypertension is shown in Figure 6.1. In its "fixed" state, hypertension involves changes in anatomic structures; that is, the medial walls of the arteries are swollen, while neurogenic vasoconstrictor discharges are minimal or normal (Folkow, 1971; Rushmer, 1970). After prolonged drug treatment, blood pressure sometimes returns to normal even after drugs are discontinued. This supports the hypothesis that hypertrophy of the medial arterial walls is reversible under conditions of reduced pressure (Folkow, 1971; Folkow, Hallback, Lundgren, Sivertsson, & Weiss, 1973).

Many investigators believe that fixed essential hypertension develops as a compensatory process in response to idiopathic high cardiac output states (Guyton, Coleman, Bower, & Granger, 1970). The process apparently develops

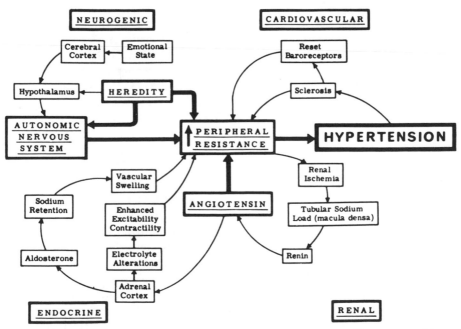

FIGURE 6.1. Possible participation of various factors in the development of hypertension. [From "Pathological physiology of the cardiovascular system. A. Hypertension" by J. J. Friedman, in E. E. Selkurt (Ed.), *Physiology* (3rd ed.) (Boston: Little, Brown, & Co.). © 1971 by Ewald E. Selkurt. Reprinted by permission.]

in genetically predisposed young adults who are cardiovascular hyperreactors under emotional or environmental stress (Eich, Cuddy, Smulyan, & Lyons, 1966; Forsyth, 1974; Frohlich, Kozul, Tarazi, & Dustan, 1970; Frohlich et al., 1969; Gorlin, Brachfeld, Turner, Messer, & Salazar, 1959; Tobian, 1972). Preventive treatment of this prehypertensive high cardiac output state may turn out to be the treatment of choice. This stage of hypertension is also known as "labile" essential hypertension, because it is often accompanied by large variability in blood pressure and/or hyperresponsiveness to stimuli of various sorts. The main physiological derangement in labile hypertension is an increased cardiac output, with or without correspondent abnormal increases in blood pressure. Total peripheral resistance often remains "abnormally normal." That is, it fails to decrease in order to compensate for the high cardiac output.

NEUROGENIC FACTORS

For a long time, informal observations and scientific evidence have led to a hypothesis that life situations and stress play a significant role in the development, maintenance, treatment, and prevention of hypertension. The evidence comes from multiple sources: anecdotal reports of patients and physicians; personality, sociological, and epidemiologic studies; psychophysiological research in humans and animals on the effects of environmental stimuli on blood pressure and other cardiovascular responses. (For reviews, see Cohen & Obrist, 1975; Eyer, 1975; Forsyth, 1974; Gutmann & Benson, 1971; Harris & Forsyth, 1973; Heine, 1971; Ostfeld & D'Atri, 1975; A. Shapiro, Redmond, McDonald, & Gaylor, 1975; A. Shapiro, Schwartz, Ferguson, Redmond, & Weiss, 1977; D. Shapiro, Mainardi, & Surwit, 1977; Stahl, Grim, Donald, & Neikirk, 1975.) Although hypertension is a very complex disorder, these data suggest that hypertension is probably initiated under the conditions of the stress of living in modern societies. Community disruption and increased work pressure are cited to be among the most important sources of this stress (Eyer, 1975). Behavioral factors interact with other determinants that increase the likelihood of developing hypertension (e.g., obesity, cigarette smoking, salt, cholesterol intake, and other dietary factors, and air and water pollutants).

If behavior has an influence on blood pressure and hypertension, the disease process must be mediated by central and autonomic nervous system mechanisms involved in the regulation of the cardiovascular system (Cohen & MacDonald, 1974; Esler et al., 1977; Forsyth, 1974; Reis, 1972). Humoral and biochemical processes are also associated with the neural and cardiovascular changes related to elevated levels of blood pressure (see Chapter 3). Little is known about the exact sequence of steps leading from behavior on the one hand to hypertension on the other, but researchers have speculated about the role of excessive sympathetic nervous system activity (Esler *et al.*, 1977) and idiopathic higher cardiac output states (Eich *et al.*, 1966; Gorlin *et al.*, 1959; Guyton *et al.*, 1970) and generally about neurogenic factors, particularly in essential hypertension. It seems likely that neurogenic hypertension represents only a part of the total population of individuals with abnormal elevations of blood pressure. Some cases of secondary hypertension may also have a neurogenic component in their etiology.

In an attempt to differentiate neurogenic from nonneurogenic hypertension, Esler *et al.* (1977) distinguished two groups of patients with mild essential hypertension: those patients who had relatively elevated levels of plasma renin activity and those with normal levels. The high renin subgroup also had a higher heart rate and an elevated plasma norepinephrine concentration. Through the use of autonomic blocking agents, these investigators established that the high renin group sustained their increased blood pressure by means of overactivity of the sympathetic nervous system. Through psychological test methods, it was learned that as a group patients with mild high renin essential hypertension were controlled, guilt prone, and submissive, had a high level of unexpressed anger, and appeared to sustain their blood pressure by means of overactivity of the sympathetic nervous system. Normal renin patients were not different from normal control subjects in these psychological characteristics. Esler *et al.* (1977) concluded that the pathogenesis of elevated blood pressure in the high renin mild hypertensive group may involve a behavioral pattern (primarily suppression of anger) that is related to increased sympathetic nervous system activity, but they also suggested that the behavior pattern could follow from increased sympathetic nervous tone rather than the other way around. Their research does not make clear why increased blood pressure is the major outcome in this group of patients (high renin) rather than some other symptom, inasmuch as excessive sympathetic nervous system activity has been believed to be a causal factor in other psychophysiological disorders as well (Shapiro & Katkin, 1980). It is not known whether the heightened sympathetic nervous tone represents a constitutional predisposition in these patients or whether the sustained and heightened sympathetic nervous tone results from repeated elicitations of behaviorally induced patterns of nervous reaction, as described in Chapter 3.

Aside from the many unresolved questions of neurogenic versus nonneurogenic hypertension, we should point out that the literature on behavioral processes in the etiology and pathogenesis of hypertension is uneven. The populations studied vary considerably according to age, sex, severity and duration of hypertension, presence of other illnesses, sociocultural factors, and so on. Variable quality of the behavioral data, incompleteness of experimental designs, and inadequacy of comparison or control groups make it difficult to interpret the significance of the studies. Granted these limitations, our aim is to begin with an overview of behavioral, social, and psychological factors in hypertension.

PERSONALITY

For many decades, attempts have been made to relate certain personality traits to a tendency to respond to emotionally arousing events with abnormal increases in blood pressure. One of the earliest characterizations of the "hypertensive personality" comes from F. Alexander (1939), who described the psychodynamics of the hypertensive patient in terms of a conflict between intense aggressive, hostile impulses and passive, dependent tendencies. Over time, the inhibition of hostile tendencies leads to a chronic elevation of blood pressure. Others have summarized the hypertensive personality as marked by a "characteristic inability to express anger, and indeed at times by an obsequious type of behavior as a retreat from potentially hostile expression [A. Shapiro *et al.*, 1975]." The presumed role of unexpressed anger in hypertension has been mentioned over and over again in the literature, although the data supporting it have not been conclusive. The research of Esler *et al.* (1977) (discussed earlier) has resurrected this hypothesis, but primarily for that subset of patients who have certain physiological characteristics (high plasma renin activity, cardiac output, etc.).

Psychological tests have been utilized in an attempt to determine if there are certain personality characteristics that are unique to hypertension. In a review of the literature, Goldstein and Shapiro (Note 1) concluded that neither projective techniques nor rating scales were able to discriminate between the behavior patterns of hypertensive and nonhypertensive patients. An exception is McClelland's (1979) report that an "inhibited power motive syndrome" (as determined from Thematic Apperception Test protocols) assessed among college undergraduates is predictive of hypertension assessed at follow-up 20 years later. Paper-and-pencil tests indicate that hypertensives tend to exhibit poor adjustment or low ego strength, characteristics associated with neurotic behavior (Harburg, Julius, McGinn, McLeod, & Hoobler, 1964; Kasl & Cobb, 1970; Pilowsky, Spalding, Shaw, & Korner, 1973). Other studies point to the hypertensive as a basically submissive individual (Hamilton, 1942; Harburg *et al.*, 1964; Pilowski *et al.*, 1973). Hypertension in black males is related to the degree of discontent they express about their social situation and a feeling of being powerless to do anything about that situation (Naditch, 1974). Hypertensive women between the ages of 45 and 64 years show a Type A coronary-prone behavior pattern, characterized by haste, aggressiveness, and excessive drive (according to the Jenkins Activity Survey) (Shekelle, Schoenberger, & Stamler,

1976). There is also evidence that a widely varying or labile blood pressure, rather than a high level of pressure, is related to a particular personality pattern of impulsivity, hypochondriasis, and hysteria according to the Minnesota Multiphasic Personality Inventory (Ostfeld & Lebovits, 1960).

Research on the hypertensive personality, if not definitive, has suggested that behavior plays a role in the disorder. The need is to translate such information on individual differences in personality traits into easily assessed behavior patterns, such as the Type A–Type B, which has been found so useful in research on heart disease (see Chapter 5). We also need to distinguish behavior patterns specifically associated with hypertension from those associated with other disorders. Which patterns are the result of being ill, and which are more causative in nature?

STRESS AND PSYCHOSOCIAL FACTORS

According to Glock and Lennard (1956, p. 179), stress "refers to an event or experience in the life of an individual which has specific physiologic consequences." These result in "disturbance in the equilibrium of the organism." While there is no evidence that stress is specific to hypertension, it has been noted that traumatic events can play a part in high blood pressure. Some illustrative data are cited.

Natural Disasters. Soldiers who spent a year in desert warfare had high blood pressure that lasted 4–8 weeks after retiring from combat (Graham, 1945). Similar instances of high blood pressure were noted during the siege of Leningrad (Miasnikov, 1962). When a ship loaded with explosive chemicals blew up a chemical plant in Texas, significant elevations in blood pressure were found. After 10–14 days, however, blood pressure returned to normal (Ruskin, Beard, & Schaffer, 1948).

Culture and Urbanization. Urban living has been associated with a variety of stressors. Individuals living in high-stress areas of Detroit (defined by low socioeconomic status, high density, high residential morbidity, and high rates of marital breakup) were found to have much higher blood pressure levels than counterparts in lower-stress areas (Harburg, Erfurt, Hauenstein, Chape, Schull, & Schork, 1973). This was particularly true for black males. D'Atri and Ostfeld (1975) found a relationship between degree of urban crowding, blood pressure, and pulse rate. Scotch (1963) found that the urban Zulus had a higher frequency of hypertension for all ages and for both sexes than rural Zulus. Hypertension was virtually nonexistent in the inhabitants of two relatively isolated Pacific islands (Maddocks, 1961). Similarly, blood pressure in two Indian tribes in Brazil was found to be low relative to other populations (Lowenstein, 1961). The frequent rise in blood pressure with age, observed in many societies, is probably a consequence of civilization and acculturation.

Cruz-Coke, Etcheverry, and Nagel (1964) introduced the concept of "ecological niche" to explain the low blood pressure among groups living in relatively isolated regions where traditions remain constant. When these people migrate to urban centers, their blood pressures rise. Both environmental changes and racial susceptibility are believed to be important. The influence of racial susceptibility may explain why Beiser, Collomb, Ravel, and Nafyigers (1976) found no evidence of an age-related rise in blood pressure for either rural or urban groups among the Serer of Senegal. Henry and Cassell (1969) concluded from a review of 18 epidemiologic studies that a failure to show a blood pressure rise with age was associated with a stable culture where tradition rather than change was important.

Occupational Stress. Constant exposure to job stresses has been a factor frequently associated with heightened blood pressure (see Mustacchi, 1977). The incidence of hypertension among air traffic controllers, whose work is very stressful, was four times greater than that among second-class airmen, who are subjected to less stress (Cobb & Rose, 1973). Those air traffic controllers who worked in high traffic density centers exhibited more cases of hypertension than did other controllers. Blood pressure levels were higher during the anticipation of job loss and unemployment than during periods of stabilization on new jobs. Individuals with the more severe unemployment experience had elevated blood pressure for the longest time periods (Kasl & Cobb, 1970).

Prolonged Illness. Heine and Sainsbury (1970) provided some evidence that prolonged depressive states were related to raised levels of blood pressure during illness. Blood pressure in an ill person tended to be correlated with the anxiety and agitation that characterized the depression. H. J. Friedman and Bennet (1977) found the diagnosis of anxiety to be significantly associated with both depression and hypertension.

EXPERIMENTALLY INDUCED STRESS

Human Studies

By means of experimental stimuli, it is possible to manipulate blood pressure levels in human beings and to show how hypertensives differ physiologically from normotensives. Ayman and Goldshine (1939) demonstrated that a breath-holding test could cause blood pressure rises from two to four times greater in hypertensive patients than in normals. In response to a cold pressor stimulus, normotensive subjects reached a maximum increase in blood pressure sooner than high and low blood pressure groups, but the hypertensives responded with far greater blood pressure increases (Thacker, 1940). During mental arithmetic performed under duress, hypertensives exhibited hemodynamic changes and blood pressure elevations that persisted longer than those exhibited by a comparison group (Brod, Fencl, Hejl, & Jurka, 1959). A delayed recovery of blood pressure to normal levels was also found by Baumann, Ziprian, Godicke, Hartrodt, Naumann, and Lauter (1973) in response to an arithmetic task.

A variety of stimuli have been utilized in human studies and have yielded relatively consistent results. Jost, Rullmann, Hill, and Gulo (1952) subjected hypertensive patients and normals to many different stimuli presented in sequence—a buzzer, a bright light, emotionally disturbing questions, and memory tests of rapidly increasing difficulty. In all parts of the experiment, hypertensives had longer-lasting blood pressure changes, which were generally in an upward direction. Cold pressor, injection of normal saline, a frustrating task, threat of electric shock, and frustration by an irritating technician all produced greater blood pressure rises in hypertensives than in control groups (Schachter, 1957; A. Shapiro, 1961). Engel and Bickford (1961) found that hypertensives would react to any stressor with a maximal blood pressure response, regardless of the stimulus.

Interview techniques have also been utilized as a mean of stimulating pressor responses in human beings. Wolff and Wolf (1951) have found that all individuals respond to topics of conflicts with rises in blood pressure, but hypertensives show much greater increases. The amount of blood pressure change depends on the meaning of the stimulus to the subject. Innes, Miller, & Valentine (1959) noted that no specific topics were associated with blood pressure increases, but blood pressure levels took longer to return to normal in hypertensives and neurotics than in controls with low blood pressure. McKegney and Williams (1967) found more pronounced and prolonged diastolic pressure increases in hypertensives than in normotensives during an interview that emphasized interpersonal interaction. Apparently, the critical factor in distinguishing hypertensives from normotensives is not just the level of response but the prolonged reaction that hypertensives have to stressful stimuli.

Animal Studies

By utilizing animals in a laboratory situation, it is possible to reproduce many environmental stressors and to manipulate the level and duration of the stimuli more precisely than is possible with human subjects. For example, it has been demonstrated that rats exposed to loud noises over long periods of time will develop signs of hypertension (Farris, Yeakel, & Medoff, 1945; Medoff & Bongiovanni, 1945; Yeakel, Shenkin, Rothballer, & McCann, 1948). Chronic intermittent exposure to auditory, visual, and motion stimuli (Smookler, Goebel, Siegel, & Clarke, 1973) as well as chronic sound withdrawal (Marwood & Lockett, 1977) induced hypertension and even produced histological changes in rats. Rats exposed to crowded cages for short periods of time experienced blood pressure elevations that reverted to normal levels in a few days. Exposures of 6 months or more were associated with more permanent blood pressure effects and with increased mortality frequently due to cerebral vascular lesions (Henry, Stephens & Santisteban, 1975).

Herd, Morse, Kelleher, and Jones (1969) are of the opinion that the presence of a noxious stimulus in itself is not enough to cause arterial pressure to increase. Operant conditioning with squirrel monkeys has led to the finding that schedules that exert strong control over an animal's behavior bring about the highest and most persistent blood pressure elevations. R. Friedman and Dahl's (1977) work with rats substantiates this finding; merely shocking rats or exposing them to food deprivation failed to result in a rise in blood pressure. Friedman and Dahl believe that exposure to conflict, especially in a strain of hypertension-susceptible rats, brings about long-lasting blood pressure increases.

Experimental evidence with human beings, as well as with lower animals, has provided sufficient evidence that stress can produce acute pressor responses. The reactions of hypertensives are generally more elevated and of a longer duration than those of normotensives. Investigations of animals have resulted in even greater blood pressure changes. Apparently, the presence of noxious stimuli has not been as effective in producing hypertension in experimental animals as the utilization of complex operant schedules where the animal is exposed to relatively long periods of conflict and continuous behavioral adjustments are required.

PHARMACOLOGIC TREATMENT OF HYPERTENSION

The current pharmacologic treatment of hypertension is based on the "stepped-care" approach.[1] When blood pressure remains consistently above 140/90 mm Hg, with repeated blood pressure determinations over the course of several weeks, the first step is to place the patient on a thiazide diuretic. This has the effect of increasing urinary excretion of sodium, as well as a direct hypotensive vasodilator effect.

[1] Report of the Joint National Committee on detection, evaluation, and treatment of high blood pressure. *Journal of the American Medical Association*, 1977, 277, 255–261.

If the diuretic does not achieve reduction of blood pressure to levels below 140/90 mm Hg, the next step is to add either a centrally acting sympatholytic agent (e.g., Methyldopa) or a beta-adrenergic blocking agent (e.g., propranolol). The latter is often used alone or along with a diuretic as the first step in patients under age 40, in whom elevated cardiac output may be more prevalent. In addition, beta blockade lessens the renin response to reduce intravascular volume due to diuretics.

If the second step does not result in normalization of blood pressure, the third step would be to add a directly acting vasodilator (e.g., hydralazine). Finally, if such triple therapy proves ineffective, guanethidine, a potent peripheral sympathetic depleter, might be substituted for methyldopa. If this proves unsuccessful, then a regimen consisting of a variety of other agents (e.g., clonidine, prazosin, etc.) must be devised on an individualized basis for each patient.

The goals of pharmacologic therapy can be conceptualized as: (*a*) decreasing blood volume, largely through promotion of increased sodium excretion, (*b*) decreasing cardiac output, largely through beta blockade, (*c*) decreasing peripheral vasoconstriction, either through the use of agents acting in the central nervous system (CNS) (e.g., methyldopa) or agents acting directly on vascular smooth muscle, and (*d*) decreasing renin secretion, through the use of beta blockade. As will be detailed in the rest of this chapter, behavioral approaches exist that can be employed, at least in an adjunctive fashion, to achieve each of these goals.

BEHAVIORAL TREATMENT OF HYPERTENSION

Biofeedback

Basic laboratory data (see Chapter 4) provide a foundation for the clinical application of biofeedback to hypertension. Benson, Shapiro, Tursky, and Schwartz (1971) used the constant-cuff technique and gave feedback and reinforcement for the lowering of systolic blood pressure in seven patients, five of whom had been diagnosed as having essential hypertension. Medication dosage, diet, and other factors were kept constant during the course of the study. Of the other two patients, one did not have elevated systolic pressure and the other had renal artery stenosis. No reductions were observed in as many as 15 pretreatment control sessions. The five patients responding positively showed decreases of 34, 29, 16, 16, and 17 mm Hg with 33, 22, 34, 31, and 12 sessions of training, respectively.

Using the same procedure, Goldman, Kleinman, Snow, Bidus, and Korol

(1975) reported average decreases of 4% and 13% in systolic and diastolic pressure, respectively, in seven patients with average baseline values of 167/ 109 mm Hg who were diagnosed as having essential hypertension and who were willing to participate in the study prior to having medication. Although feedback was given for systolic pressure, the significant reductions occurred only in diastolic pressure over the course of the nine training sessions. Those patients who showed greatest decreases in both systolic and diastolic pressure during biofeedback training also showed the greatest improvement on the category test of the Halstead–Reitan Neuropsychological Test Battery for Adults (Reitan, 1966). The results may imply that biofeedback may be useful in lowering pressure *and* in overcoming a cognitive impairment associated with hypertension (Reitan, 1954; Richter-Heinrich & Läuter, 1969). Moreover, the improvement in cognitive functioning suggests that the effects of biofeedback training may not be entirely laboratory specific.

Miller (1975) attempted to train 28 patients with essential hypertension to reduce their diastolic blood pressure. A few patients appeared to reduce their blood pressure, but after reaching a plateau, the pressure drifted up again. One patient showing good results was trained to alternately increase and decrease her pressure. Over a period of 3 months, this patient acquired the ability to change pressure over a range of 30 mm Hg. Her baseline pressure decreased from 97 to 76 mm Hg, and similar decreases were observed on the ward; medication was discontinued. Later on, she lost voluntary control as a result of life stresses and was put back on drugs. When the patient came back to training 2.5 years later, she rapidly regained a large measure of control. Such multiple courses of treatment may facilitate relatively permanent "cures."

Kristt and Engel (1975) reported evidence that patients with essential hypertension having a variety of cardiovascular and other complications can learn to control and reduce their pressure over and above the effects produced by drugs. In phase 1, the patients took their pressure at home daily over a 7-week period and mailed in their reports to the laboratory. In phase 2, patients were trained to raise, to lower, and to alternately raise and lower systolic blood pressure using the constant-cuff method (see Chapter 2). In phase 3, the patients again took their pressure at home and mailed in daily reports. Learned control of pressure was observed in all patients during the training sessions, and reductions in pressure of about 10–15% were observed from pretraining baselines to values recorded at a 3-month follow-up. Although feedback training was provided for systolic pressure, diastolic pressure was also reduced.

Since systolic blood pressure has been found to be more associated than diastolic pressure with morbidity and mortality in males over 45 years of age, reductions in systolic pressure could be a treatment of choice for this particular age–sex population. Also, morbidity and mortality in females seem to be more dependent upon systolic than diastolic pressure at almost all ages (Kannel *et al.*,

1971). In younger men, diastolic pressure is more closely associated with morbidity and mortality (Kannel *et al.*, 1971), in agreement with traditional concepts of hypertension (Merrill, 1966). Diastolic pressure is thought to be more critical in later or final states of hypertension because of its closer relation to peripheral resistance (Merrill, 1966). Preliminary research (Benson, Shapiro, & Schwartz, Note 2) suggests that it is difficult to reduce abnormally high diastolic levels in patients with hypertension (Schwartz & Shapiro, 1973). Part of the problem may be related to unreliability in obtaining consistent diastolic values over repeated sessions. Learned control of diastolic pressure was observed in a single-session study of normal subjects, with consistent changes occurring in almost all subjects (D. Shapiro, Schwartz, & Tursky, 1972). However, positive results in biofeedback training in patients with decreases in diastolic pressure have been reported in other laboratories. Using feedback and verbal praise, 20–30% reductions in diastolic pressure were obtained in patients diagnosed as essential hypertensives (Elder, Ruiz, Deabler, & Dillenkoffer, 1973). None of the 18 patients studied were under antihypertensive medication, although many were on CNS depressants.

Surwit, Shapiro, and Good (1978) reported findings of a controlled group outcome study in which two types of biofeedback training were compared to a form of meditation in the treatment of borderline hypertension. Twenty-four borderline hypertensives served as subjects and were evenly divided into three treatment conditions. All subjects received two 1-hr baseline sessions and eight 1-hr biweekly treatment sessions. The first treatment group received binary feedback for simultaneous reductions of blood pressure and heart rate (Schwartz, Shapiro, & Tursky, 1972). The second group received analog feedback for combined forearm and frontalis electromyographic (EMG) activity. The third group received a meditation–relaxation procedure (Benson, 1975). Six weeks following the last treatment session, all subjects received a 1-hr treatment follow-up session. Data analysis indicated that the three treatment groups all showed significant reductions in pressure over trials during each session, implying that each of the behavioral methods tested was equally effective as a clinical intervention. Carry-over effects from session to session or in a 1-year follow-up were not significant. Borderline or labile patients revealed normal pressure levels in a quiet laboratory, suggesting that such conditions may not be appropriate for relearning. High levels of pressure may be under the control of particular situational events, and patients would therefore need to learn to reduce their reactivity in relation to such triggering stimuli.

In another group outcome study, Walsh, Dale, and Anderson (1977) and Dale, Anderson, Walsh, and Weiss (1978) compared biofeedback for pulse transit time (PTT) against progressive relaxation in reducing blood pressure. In a study of 24 hypertensive patients, they found that progressive relaxation was superior to PTT feedback within each session. However, patients receiving

PTT feedback showed the greatest reduction in a 3-month follow-up: PTT feedback, 151/94 mm Hg to 133/85 mm Hg; progressive relaxation, 142/92 mm Hg to 146/91 mm Hg. In a 1-year follow-up, the PTT and progressive relaxation conditions did not differ. The authors concluded that progressive relaxation may be cheaper and more practical than PTT feedback training.

Some of the studies reviewed using direct blood pressure feedback and pulse wave velocity feedback have reported that heart rate changes did not seem to be related to learned changes in systolic blood pressure and pulse wave velocity. Since cardiac output is in part a function of heart rate, one might speculate that successful subjects were reducing blood pressure by reducing peripheral resistance. Since blood pressure is maintained through a homeostatic interplay between cardiac output and peripheral resistance, it is possible that blood pressure feedback or pulse wave velocity feedback may result in compensatory changes in cardiac output and thereby limit pressure change. Williams (1975) concluded that a more effective means of reducing blood pressure would be to give feedback for reductions in both cardiac output and peripheral resistance. Williams treated a single patient diagnosed as essential hypertensive (mean blood pressure = 200/130 mm Hg), whose blood pressure was difficult to control because of disturbing drug side effects. Assuming that heart rate relates to cardiac output and forearm blood flow to peripheral resistance, Williams gave the patient 5 days of training for simultaneous reductions of heart rate and increases in forearm blood flow. Blood pressure was also recorded using the standard cuff method. Williams reported substantial control of heart rate and forearm blood flow. Blood pressure declined from 164/124 mm Hg to 143/116 mm Hg over the 5 days of training, with a 4-month follow-up ranging from 160–150/110–105 mm Hg, including the effects of sympatholytic and diuretic drug treatment. The hypothesis was supported that combined feedback of two cardiovascular parameters to achieve peripheral vasodilatation without compensatory increases in cardiac output can produce clinically significant decreases in both systolic and diastolic blood pressure.

Several investigators attempted to reduce blood pressure by giving biofeedback for physiological activity assumed to influence or mediate blood pressure indirectly. Based on research showing that progressive relaxation (Jacobson, 1939) and autogenic training (Luthe & Schultz, 1969) can reliably reduce blood pressure, Moeller and Love (Note 3) undertook to investigate the clinical effectiveness of biofeedback for reduced EMG activity to achieve relaxation in a group of six hypertensive patients (mean blood pressure = 153/110 mm Hg). Frontal (frontalis muscle area) EMG biofeedback was combined with autogenic training for 17 sessions. The investigators reported average blood pressure reductions of 18/12 mm Hg. Moeller (1973) obtained similar results in a sample of 36 patients given the same procedures. Love, Montgomery, and Moeller (Note 4) extended these findings. Forty essential hypertensive patients (mean blood pressure = 162/106 mm Hg) received 16 weeks of either frontal EMG biofeedback plus taped autogenic training, EMG biofeedback and no autogenic training, or control sessions in which frontal EMG was recorded. The treatment groups did not differ and showed average decreases of 15/13 mm Hg. The control group showed no pressure changes. An 8-month follow-up showed even further pressure reductions of 6.5/4 mm Hg. These studies suggest that frontal EMG biofeedback alone, or in combination with autogenic training, may provide an effective treatment for hypertensive patients. The procedure has a possible advantage in that patients may be more likely to be able to sense and control their muscles (proprioceptive feedback) and thereby possibly develop a means of self-control of blood pressure outside the laboratory. Recall, however, that Surwit *et al.* (1978) failed to obtain blood pressure reductions in patients given EMG biofeedback for two muscles. In addition, A. B. Alexander (1975) questioned the effectiveness of frontal EMG biofeedback as a means of producing general relaxation.

Probably the most impressive clinical results were reported by Patel (1977). Based on the widely held assumption that excessive sympathetic nervous system activity plays a role in the etiology and maintenance of hypertension, Patel proposed to modify sympathetic activity by using skin resistance biofeedback. Patel (1973) combined biofeedback for increasing skin resistance with a form of yoga breathing–relaxation exercise and a passive concentration or meditation to treat a group of 20 hypertensive patients. Initial average blood pressure on medication was 160/102 mm Hg. Following 36 half-hour sessions over a 3-month period, average pressure dropped to 134/86 mm Hg. Furthermore, total drug requirement was reduced by 41.9%. Only four patients failed to demonstrate improvement. Patel (1975a) compared 20 patients from her first study with an age–sex matched control group in order to assess the effects of increased medical attention and repeated blood pressure measurements on blood pressure reductions. Controls were also instructed to rest quietly for 30 min on a couch in the hospital. After a 12-month follow-up period, the treatment group had average pressure reductions of 20.4/14.2 mm Hg compared to no change for the controls. Patel and North (1975) attempted to establish the scientific validity of the treatment procedure by randomly assigning patients to either a treatment or a control group. Although the treatment procedure was similar to the one used in Patel's previous studies, frontal EMG biofeedback was also employed. Controls attended the same number of sessions during which they were asked to relax. The number of treatment sessions was reduced to 2 sessions per week for 6 weeks. A 3-month follow-up was recorded. Systolic blood pressure fell an average of 26.1 mm Hg for the treatment group and 8.9 mm Hg for the control group. Respective reductions in diastolic blood pressure were 15.2 mm Hg and 4.2 mm Hg. These differences were highly significant. Thus, the substantial reductions reported by Patel seem to reflect a multimodal behavioral treatment regime and not attention placebo or nonspecific effects. Moreover, Patel (1975b) also demonstrated that patients were less reactive to exercise and cold pressor tests following treatment than were controls. What role skin resistance or EMG biofeedback play in reducing pressure, however, is impossible to ascertain, since relaxation was always combined with biofeedback.

Relaxation and Other Techniques

Jacob, Kraemer, and Agras (1977) provided a conprehensive review of the use of relaxation training in the treatment of hypertension. The relaxation approaches have used variations of either certain Eastern meditative disciplines, progressive relaxation as developed by Jacobson (1939), or autogenic training, pioneered by Schultz and Luthe (1969). These techniques are intended to lower blood pressure by promoting physical and mental relaxation. Benson, Rosner, Marzetta, and Klemchuk (1974a,b) used a procedure derived from transcendental meditation (Mahesh Yogi, 1966) to produce a hypometabolic state termed the *relaxation response* (Benson, 1975; Benson, Benary, & Carol, 1974). The method was used in a study of 22 untreated borderline hypertensive patients and 14 pharmacologically treated hypertensive patients. The procedure involves having the patient close his eyes and silently say the word *one* during each exhalation. Maintenance of a "passive attitude" is emphasized. Mean blood pressure during a 6-week baseline was 147/95 mm Hg for the untreated borderline hypertensives and 146/92 mm Hg for the pharmacologically treated patients. Following 20–25 weeks of meditation–relaxation, blood pressure reductions of 8/4 mm Hg and 11/5 mm Hg were reported for the borderline and pharmacologic groups, respectively. These results were replicated by Blackwell, Bloomfield, Gartside, Robinson, Hanenson, Magenheim, Nidich, and Zigler (1976).

Using a similar Buddhist meditation–relaxation procedure, Stone and DeLeo (1976) reported small but significant pressure reductions from a baseline of 146/95 mm Hg to 131/85 mm Hg in 19 patients over a 6-month period. Moreover significant reductions in plasma dopamine-beta-hydroxylase activity and furosemide-stimulated plasma renin activity were found. No changes were reported in a no-treatment control group. Stone and DeLeo concluded that decreased peripheral adrenergic activity may be associated with the reduction of blood pressure resulting from the regular practice of meditation–relaxation. Datey, Deshmukh, Dalvi, and Vinekar (1969) used a yogic exercise called Shavasan to treat 47 hypertensive patients with mixed diagnoses. The exercise also focused on slow breathing and was performed daily for a 40-week period. Ten patients not under antihypertensive drugs reduced their blood pressure an average of 37/23 mm Hg from their pretreatment pressure of 185/109 mm Hg. In another sample of 22 patients whose pressures were stabilized with medications (mean blood pressure = 137/86 mm Hg), drug dosage requirements were reduced by 32% in 13 of the 22 patients. Finally, in a third group of 15 patients whose blood pressures were not adequately controlled by medications, blood pressure was reduced from an average of 167/105 mm Hg to 158/96 mm Hg. Six of these patients also reduced their dosage requirements by 29%. Overall, 65% of the patients diagnosed as essential hypertensives responded favorably to this treatment, as did 42% of the renal hypertensives. However, the three patients with arteriosclerotic hypertension failed to respond to treatment. All together, 25 of the 47 patients benefited from the yogic exercise.

Based on Jacobson's (1939) early research on the relationship between muscle tension and blood pressure, Graham, Beiman, and Ciminero (1977) treated a case of essential hypertension using progressive relaxation. This well-conducted, systematic case study reported a substantial reduction of blood pressure into the normotensive range after 25 days of training. The pressure reduction generalized outside the laboratory and even to stressful life situations. Brady, Luborsky, and Kron (1974) reported reliable diastolic blood pressure reductions from an average of 90.1 mm Hg to 86.7 mm Hg in four hypertensive patients following metronome-conditioned relaxation. This procedure involved pairing the rhythmic beats of the metronome set of 60 per minute with taped recordings of suggestions to "re-lax" and "let-go" of the muscles. The pressure reductions, however, occurred only during the training session. Two of the patients did show further diastolic pressure reductions after using the tape recordings at home.

Taylor, Farquhar, Nelson, and Agras (1977) conducted a controlled outcome study comparing a standardized tape-recorded progressive relaxation program to a "plausible alternative psychological treatment" and a medication-only treatment group. The alternative treatment consisted of five 30-min sessions of nondirective therapy aimed at encouraging patients to identify and deal with life stress. Following an average of five weekly 30-min sessions, the 11 patients in the relaxation group reduced their blood pressure from an average of 150/96 mm Hg to 137/91 mm Hg. The nondirective therapy group reduced its pressure readings from 141/90 mm Hg to 130/88.4 mm Hg, with no substantial changes for the medication group (mean blood pressure = 146/96 mm Hg). The relaxation group had statistically significantly better systolic blood pressure reductions and marginally reliable diastolic blood pressure reductions when compared to the nondirective therapy group. This group utilized an important control for nonspecific expectation factors not addressed by no-treatment control groups.

Luthe (1963) reported good blood pressure reductions using autogenic training. The procedure involves self-suggestions of warmth, passivity, and total bodily relaxation and is aimed at producing physical and psychological relaxation. Klumbies and Eberhardt (1966) reported average decreases of 35/18 mm Hg in 26 of 83 hypertensive patients also using autogenic training.

Hypnosis has also been used to treat hypertension. Deabler, Fidel, Dillenkoffer, and Elder (1973) gave 15 hypertensive patients nine sessions consisting first of progressive relaxation followed by a hypnotic induction to relax their mind and body. Six of the patients were not being treated pharmacologically (mean blood pressure = 163/96 mm Hg) and 9 patients were taking antihypertensive medications (mean blood pressure = 158/95 mm Hg). A control group that used blood pressure measurement only was also employed (mean blood pressure = 155/95 mm Hg). Mean percentage blood pressure reductions from baseline for the nonmedicated subjects was 10.5–10.6% with relaxation and 16–16.3% with relaxation plus hypnosis. The patients taking antihypertensives showed similar results, with no changes occurring for the control group. While relaxation plus hypnosis consistently resulted in lower pressures than did relaxation only, the results were confounded by an order effect. That is, relaxation plus hypnosis always followed relaxation during the treatment sessions.

In another experiment, H. Friedman and Taub (1977) compared a noncontinuous form of diastolic blood pressure feedback with hypnosis only, a diastolic blood pressure feedback plus hypnosis, and a measurement-only control group. Following seven sessions of training, significant reductions on a 1-month follow-up were found in the hypnosis-only group, from 142.5/93.1 mm Hg to 131.9/86.1 mm Hg, and in the group using diastolic blood pressure feedback only, from 146.5/95.8 mm Hg to 136.9/93.5 mm Hg. The hypnosis plus biofeedback reported smaller reductions, from 139.8/91.8 mm Hg to 139.5/86 mm Hg. The measurement-only controls showed no substantial changes from their baseline pressure of 140/95 mm Hg. A 6-month follow-up (H. Friedman & Taub, 1978) produced similar results. When all groups were compared, only the hypnosis-only group reliably differed from the control group. The authors concluded that, while diastolic blood pressure feedback only is capable of effecting pressure reductions, "hypnosis enjoys some advantage over other procedures as an effective technique for lowering blood pressure [p. 343]." These conclusions, however, should be tempered because of methodological problems. H. Friedman and Taub (1977, 1978) used only high susceptible patients in their two hypnosis groups and low susceptibles in the biofeedback-only and control groups. Thus, the experimental groups were made up of different populations. In addition, as has been discussed previously, the effectiveness of noncontinuous blood pressure feedback, such as employed by Friedman and Taub, is questionable.

Frankel, Patel, Horwitz, Friedewald, and Gaarder (1978) used several techniques in the treatment of essential hypertension. Blood pressure feedback was combined with EMG feedback and autogenic and relaxation training during 20 laboratory sessions. There was no signficant drop in blood pressure in the experimental group as compared with the patients receiving either sham or active treatment. However, most of the patients in the active group reported an increased ability to relax and to cope more effectively with stress. The authors allude to the frustration that may have resulted because the patients were unsuccessful in coping with the combined demands of blood pressure and EMG feedback. A valuable part of the study was the inclusion of an assessment of blood pressure by a nurse who was blind to the patient's experimental status. The nurse instructed the patients to relax generally but not to practice their techniques while blood pressures were being recorded. It is possible that the results of this procedure were complicated by the nurse telling the patients *not* to do what they had previously been taught to do in the laboratory.

Ongoing research at UCLA (D. Shapiro, I. Goldstein, M. Sambhi, and collaborators) has involved a comparative evaluation of drug and behavioral treatments in patients with mild to moderate essential hypertension. The two behavioral treatments were the relaxation response (Benson, Beary, & Carol, 1974) and blood pressure biofeedback (D. Shapiro, Tursky, Gershon, & Stern, 1969). These behavioral treatments were given to patients not being treated with drugs. The drug group included patients mainly treated with diuretics. A fourth group was studied as a control. These were also unmedicated patients who monitored their own blood pressure daily and participated in the same measurement and evaluation sessions as the other patients. The analyses of this 4-year study are still in progress. Preliminary analysis indicates that biweekly sessions of 8 weeks' duration of blood pressure biofeedback are more effective than the relaxation response but not as effective as drugs in reducing blood pressure (see Table 6.1).

The comparability of blood pressure reduction for drugs and biofeedback was revealed primarily in laboratory measurements and not in home recordings. The self-monitoring control group showed little reduction in blood pressure, about the same change as the relaxation response group. The decreases observed in basal blood pressures were also reflected during exposure to mental stress (mental arithmetic) and pain (cold pressor test). Although the particular relaxation exercise used in this study (relaxation response) failed to reduce the blood pressures of patients, the fact that most patients in the biofeedback group were utilizing some form of relaxation in addition to biofeedback as a means of reducing blood pressure further emphasizes the potential effectiveness of both relaxation and biofeedback in controlling the blood pressure of hypertensives.

These data suggest that although drug treatment is consistent in its effectiveness, a behavioral procedure can also be effective in reducing blood pressure

TABLE 6.1
Summary of Blood Pressure Changes from Baseline to End of Treatment[a]

	Systolic blood pressure				Diastolic blood pressure			
	RL	BF	DR	SM	RL	BF	DR	SM
Laboratory data								
No change or increase	6	3	1	5	7	2	2	5
1–4 mm Hg decrease	2	1	1	2	1	3	2	3
5–9 mm Hg decrease	0	3	1	1	1	3	3	1
10–14 mm Hg decrease	0	0	2	1	0	1	1	0
> 14 mm Hg decrease	1	2	4	0	0	0	1	0
Home A.M. data								
No change or increase	6	3	0	5	5	3	0	6
1–4 mm Hg decrease	2	2	0	2	3	3	2	3
5–9 mm Hg decrease	1	1	2	1	1	0	2	0
10–14 mm Hg decrease	0	0	4	1	0	2	2	0
> 14 mm Hg decrease	0	2	3	0	0	0	3	0
Home P.M. data								
No change or increase	7	4	0	2	3	2	0	4
1–4 mm Hg decrease	0	0	0	4	4	3	1	5
5–9 mm Hg decrease	2	2	1	3	1	1	3	0
10–14 mm Hg decrease	0	0	2	0	1	2	3	0
> 14 mm Hg decrease	0	2	6	0	0	0	2	0

[a] RL = relaxation treatment; BF = biofeedback treatment; DR = drug treatment; SM = self-monitoring control.

in some, if not all, patients (without medication). Thus, the use of drug and behavioral treatment combined could be beneficial for many patients and could lessen drug requirements.

CONCLUSION

Research on the regulation of high blood pressure by behavioral methods has produced results suggesting their clinical potential. In a number of different laboratories and hospitals and in a variety of different patients, positive results have been obtained in many if not all, studies. As a whole, however, the evidence is not conclusive, given the relatively small total number of patients treated, the lack of long-term follow-up studies, the incomplete medical and physiological evaluation of the effects of behavioral treatments, the unsystematic selection of patients, and the failure to compare different specific treatments with one another and with no-treatment or placebo control groups. Considering the long history of attempts to manage hypertension through behavioral and psychological procedures and recent successes with such methods, and considering the potential significance of nonpharmacologic approaches to hypertension, research on the problem merits a great deal more attention.

Since biofeedback and relaxation techniques have by and large resulted in equivalent blood pressure reductions, the less costly and simpler relaxation procedures may be the treatment of choice. The combination of biofeedback and relaxation has produced the most substantial pressure reductions. However, studies combining biofeedback and relaxation have employed designs that make it impossible to assess the relative contributions of each method to such reductions. Research addressing whether biofeedback itself adds anything unique over and above simpler relaxation techniques is needed.

Another approach would be to attempt to match behavioral treatment and individual patients according to the patient's characteristics. The treatment might be dictated by a careful medical and psychophysiological analysis of the patient under resting and stressful circumstances. Esler *et al.* (1977) have shown that some borderline and mild to moderate cases of hypertension may be characterized as having heightened sympathetic nervous system activity, as indicated by elevated levels of plasma renin activity, catecholamines, cardiac output, and other indexes. A general relaxation technique aimed at reducing sympathetic nervous tone might be most effective with such patients. Patients with fixed hypertension may benefit less than patients who are labile.

In conclusion, behavioral procedures are attractive in that they might provide alternative or adjunctive modalities in the treatment of high blood pressure, thereby increasing patient compliance and satisfaction and possibly increasing the effectiveness of drug therapy. Continued further research and clinical experiences will bring us still closer to converting biofeedback and other behavioral approaches into accepted medical practice. This research requires close collaboration between physicians, behavioral scientists, physiologists, and biochemists, so that particular applications and evaluations of behavioral methods can evolve along more productive and more comprehensive lines. Through interdisciplinary efforts in appropriate clinical and medical settings, this area of research should prove to have significant practical value for the treatment of hypertension and for our understanding of the disorder itself and of interactions between environmental demands, behavior, and the cardiovascular system.

REFERENCE NOTES

1. Goldstein, I. B., & Shapiro, D. The relationship between personality tests and blood pressure. Unpublished paper.

2. Benson, H., Shapiro, D., & Schwartz, G. E. Unpublished data, 1972.
3. Moeller, T. A., & Love, W. A. A method to reduce arterial hypertension through muscular relaxation. Unpublished manuscript, Nova University, Fort Lauderdale, Florida, 1974.
4. Love, W. A., Montgomery, D. D., & Moeller, T. A. Working Paper No. 1. Unpublished manuscript, Nova University, Fort Lauderdale, Florida, 1974.

REFERENCES

Alexander, A. B. An experimental test of assumptions relating to the use of electromyographic biofeedback as a general relaxation technique. *Psychophysiology,* 1975, *12,* 656–662.
Alexander, F. Psychoanalytic study of a case of essential hypertension. *Psychosomatic Medicine,* 1939 *1,* 139–152.
Ayman, D., & Goldshine, A. D. The breath-holding test: A simple standard stimulus of blood pressure. *Archives of Internal Medicine,* 1939, *63,* 899–906.
Baumann, R., Ziprian, H., Godicke, W., Hartrodt, W., Naumann, E., & Läuter, J. The influence of acute psychic stress situations on biochemical and vegetative parameters of essential hypertensives at the early stage of the disease. *Psychotherapy and Psychosomatics,* 1973, *22,* 131–140.
Beiser, M., Collomb, H., Ravel, J.-L., & Nafyigers, C. J. Systemic blood pressure studies among the Serer of Senegal. *Journal of Chronic Diseases,* 1976, *29,* 371–380.
Benson, H. *The relaxation response.* New York: Morrow, 1975.
Benson, H., Beary, J. F., & Carol, M. P. The relaxation response. *Psychiatry,* 1974, *37,* 37–46.
Benson, H., Rosner, B. A., Marzetta, B. R., & Klemchuk, H. P. Decreased blood pressure in borderline hypertensive subjects who practiced meditation. *Journal of Chronic Disease,* 1974, *27,* 163–169. (a)
Benson, H., Rosner, B. A., Marzetta, B. R., & Klemchuk, H. P. Decreased blood pressure in pharmacologically treated hypertensive patients who regularly elicited the relaxation response. *Lancet,* 1974, *7852,* 289–291. (b)
Benson, H., Shapiro, D., Tursky, B., & Schwartz, G. E. Decreased systolic blood pressure through operant conditioning techniques in patients with essential hypertension. *Science,* 1971, *173,* 740–742.
Blackwell, B., Bloomfield, S., Gartside, P., Robinson, A., Hanenson, I., Magenheim, H., Nidich, S., & Zigler, R. Transcendental meditation in hypertension: Individual response patterns. *Lancet,* 1976, *7953,* 223–226.
Brady, J. B., Luborsky, L., & Kron, R. E. Blood pressure reduction in patients with essential hypertension through metrone-conditioned relaxation: A preliminary report. *Behavior Therapy,* 1974, *5,* 203–209.
Brod, J. Circulation in muscle during acute pressor responses to emotional stress and during chronic sustained elevation of blood pressure. *American Heart Journal,* 1964, *68,* 424–426.
Brod, J., Fencl, V., Hejl, Z., & Jurka, J. Circulatory changes underlying blood pressure elevation during acute emotional stress (mental arithmetic) in normotensive and hypertensive subjects. *Clinical Science,* 1959, *18,* 269–279.
Bunag, R. D., Page, I. H., & McCubbin, J. W. Neural stimulation of release of renin. *Circulation Research,* 1966, *19,* 851–858.
Cobb, S., & Rose, E. M. Hypertension, peptic ulcer and diabetes in air traffic controllers. *Journal of the American Medical Association,* 1973, *224,* 489–492.
Cohen, D. H., & MacDonald, R. L. A selective review of central neural pathways involved in cardiovascular control. In P. A. Obrist, A. H. Black, J. Brener, & L. V. DiCara (Eds.), *Cardiovascular psychophysiology.* Chicago: Aldine, 1974.

Cohen, D. H., & Obrist, P. A. Interactions between behavior and the cardiovascular system. *Circulation Research*, 1975, *37*, 693–706.

Cruz-Coke, R., Etcheverry, R., & Nagel, R. Influence of migration on blood pressure of Easter islanders. *Lancet*, 1964, *1169*, 695–699.

Dale, A., Anderson, D. E., Walsh, P., & Weiss, S. Mediating mechanisms in the biofeedback control of arterial pulse wave velocity. *Psychophysiology*, 1978, *15*, 266. (Abstract)

Datey, K. K., Deshmukh, S. N., Dalvi, C. P., & Vinekar, S. L. "Shavasan": A yogic exercise in the management of hypertension. *Angiology*, 1969, *20*, 325–333.

D'Atri, D. A., & Ostfeld, A. M. Crowding: Its effects on the elevation of blood pressure in a prison setting. *Preventive Medicine*, 1975, *4*, 550–566.

Davis, J. O. What signals the kidney to release renin? *Circulation Research*, 1971, *28*, 301–306.

Deabler, H. L., Fidel, E., Dillenkoffer, R. L., & Elder, S. T. The use of relaxation and hypnosis in lowering high blood pressure. *American Journal of Clinical Hypnosis*, 1973, *16*, 75–83.

DeQuattro, V., & Miura, V. Neurogenic factors in human hypertension: Mechanism or myth? *American Journal of Medicine*, 1973, *55*, 362–378.

Dustan, H. P., Tarazi, R. C., & Bravo, E. L. Physiologic characteristics of hypertension. *American Journal of Medicine*, 1972, *52*, 610–622.

Eich, R. H., Cuddy, R. P., Smulyan, H. L., & Lyons, R. H. Haemodynamics in labile hypertension. *Circulation*, 1966, *34*, 299–307.

Elder, S. T., Ruiz, Z. R., Deabler, H. L., & Dillenkoffer, R. L. Instrumental conditioning of diastolic blood pressure in essential hypertensive patients. *Journal of Applied Behavior Analysis*, 1973, *6*, 377–382.

Engel, B. T., & Bickford, A. F. Response specificity: Stimulus-response and individual-response specificity in essential hypertensives. *Archives of General Psychiatry*, 1961, *5*, 478–489.

Esler, M., Julius, S., Zweifler, A., Randall, O., Harburg, E., Gardiner, H., & DeQuattro, V. Mild high-renin essential hypertension: Neurogenic human hypertension? *New England Journal of Medicine*, 1977, *296*, 405–411.

Eyer, J. Hypertension as a disease of modern society. *International Journal of Health Services*, 1975, *5*, 539–558.

Farris, E. J., Yeakel, E. H., & Medoff, H. S. Development of hypertension in emotional gray Norway rats after air blasting. *American Journal of Physiology*, 1945, *144*, 331–333.

Folkow, B. Regulation of the peripheral circulation. *American Heart Journal*, 1971, *33* (Suppl.), 27–31.

Folkow, B., Hallback, M., Lundgren, Y., Silvertsson, R., & Weiss, L. Importance of adaptive changes in vascular design for establishment of primary hypertension, studied in man and in spontaneously hypertensive rats. *Circulation Research*, 1973, *32* (Suppl. 1), 12–16.

Folkow, B., & Rubinstein, E. H. Cardiovascular effects of acute and chronic stimulations of the hypothalamic defense area in the rat. *Acta Physiologica Scandinavia*, 1966, *68*, 48–57.

Forsyth, R. P. Mechanisms of the cardiovascular responses to environmental stressors. In P. A. Obrist, A. H. Black, J. Brener, & L. V. DiCara (Eds.), *Cardiovascular psychophysiology*. Chicago: Aldine, 1974.

Frankel, B. L., Patel, D. J., Horwitz, D., Friedewald, W. T., & Gaarder, K. R. Treatment of hypertension with biofeedback and relaxation techniques. *Psychosomatic Medicine*, 1978, *40*, 276–293.

Freis, E. D. The clinical spectrum of essential hypertension. *Archives of Internal Medicine*, 1974, *133*, 982–987.

Friedman, H., & Taub, H. A. The use of hypnosis and biofeedback procedures for essential hypertension. *International Journal of Clinical and Experimental Hypnosis*, 1977, *25*, 335–347.

Friedman, H., & Taub, H. A. A six-month follow-up of the use of hypnosis and biofeedback procedures in essential hypertension. *American Journal of Clinical Hypnosis*, 1978, *20*, 184–188.

Friedman, M. J., & Bennet, P. L. Depression and hypertension. *Psychosomatic Medicine,* 1977, *39,* 134–142.

Friedman, R., & Dahl, L. K. The effect of chronic conflict in the blood pressure of rats with a genetic susceptibility to experimental hypertension. In D. Wheatly (Ed.), *Stress and the heart.* New York: Raven, 1977.

Frohlich, E. D., Kozul, V. J., Tarazi, R. C., & Dustan, H. P. Physiological comparison of labile and essential hypertension. *Circulation Research,* 1970, *27* (Suppl. 1), 155–163.

Frohlich, E. D., Tarazi, R. C., & Dustan, H. P. Re-examination of the hemodynamics of hypertension. *American Journal of Medical Sciences,* 1969, *257,* 9–23.

Frohlich, E. D., Ulrych, M., Tarazi, R. C., Dustan, H. P., & Page. I. H. A hemodynamic comparison of essential and renovascular hypertension. *Circulation,* 1967, *35,* 289–297.

Glock, C. Y., & Lennard, H. L. Studies in hypertension. V: Psychologic factors in hypertension: An interpretive review. *Journal of Chronic Diseases,* 1956, *5,* 174–185.

Goldman, H., Kleinman, K. M., Snow, M. Y., Bidus, D. R., & Korol, B. Relationship between essential hypertension and cognitive functioning: Effects of biofeedback. *Psychophysiology,* 1975, *12,* 569–573.

Gorlin, R., Brachfeld, N., Turner, J. D., Messer, J. V., & Salazar, E. The idiopathic high cardiac output state. *Journal of Clinical Investigation,* 1959, *38,* 2144–2153.

Graham, J. D. P. High blood pressure after battle, *Lancet,* 1945, 239–240.

Graham, L. E., Beiman, I., & Ciminero, A. R. The generality of the therapeutic effects of progressive relaxation training for essential hypertension. *Journal of Behavior Therapy and Experimental Psychiatry,* 1977, *8,* 161–164.

Gutmann, M. C., & Benson, H. Interaction of environmental factors and systemic arterial blood pressure: A review. *Medicine,* 1971, *50,* 543–553.

Guyton, A. C., Coleman, T. G., Bower, J. D., & Granger, H. J. Circulatory control in hypertension. *Circulation Research,* 1970, *26* (Suppl. 2), 135–147.

Hamilton, J. A. Psychophysiology of blood pressure. *Psychosomatic Medicine,* 1942, *4,* 125–133.

Harburg, E., Erfurt, J. C., Hauenstein, L. S., Chape, C., Schull, W. J., & Schork, M. A. Socio-ecological stress, suppressed hostility, skin color, and black–white male blood pressure: Detroit. *Psychosomatic Medicine,* 1973, *35,* 276–296.

Harburg, E., Julius, S., McGinn, N. F., McLeod, J., & Hoobler, S. W. Personality traits and behavioral patterns associated with systolic blood pressure levels in college males. *Journal of Chronic Diseases,* 1964, *17,* 405–414.

Harris, R. E., & Forsyth, R. P. Personality and emotional stress in essential hypertension in man. In G. Onesti, K. E. Kim, & J. H. Moyer (Eds.), *Hypertension: Mechanisms and management.* New York: Grune & Stratton, 1973.

Heine, B. Psychosomatic aspects of hypertension. *Postgraduate Medical Journal,* 1971, *47,* 541– 548.

Heine, B., & Sainsbury, P. Prolonged emotional disturbance and essential hypertension. *Psychotherapy and Psychosomatics,* 1970, *18,* 341–348.

Henry, J. P., & Cassel, J. C. Psychosocial factors in essential hypertension: Recent epidemiological and animal experimental evidence. *American Journal of Epidemiology,* 1969, *90,* 171–200.

Henry, J. P., Stephens, P. M., & Santisteban, G. A. A model of psychosocial hypertension showing reversibility and progression of cardiovascular complications. *Circulation Research,* 1975, *36,* 156–164.

Herd, J. A., Morse, W. H., Kelleher, R. T., & Jones, L. G. Arterial hypertension in the squirrel monkey during behavioral experiments. *American Journal of Physiology,* 1969, *217,* 24–29.

Hypertension Detection and Follow-up Program Cooperative Group, 1979. Five year findings of the Hypertension Detection and Follow-up Program. I. Reduction in mortality of persons with high blood pressure, including mild hypertension. *Journal of American Medical Association*, 1979, *242*, 2562–2571.

Innes, G., Miller, W. M., & Valentine, M. Emotion and blood pressure. *Journal of Medical Science*, 1959, *105*, 840–851.

Jacob, R. G., Kramer, H. C., & Agras, S. Relaxation therapy in the treatment of hypertension. A review. *Archives of General Psychiatry*, 1977, *34*, 1417–1427.

Jacobson, E. Variation of blood pressure with skeletal muscle tension and relaxation. *Annals of Internal Medicine*, 1939, *12*, 1194–1212.

Jost, H., Rullmann, C. J., Hill, T. S., & Gulo, M. J. Studies in hypertension: II. Central and autonomic nervous system reactions of hypertensive individuals to simple physical and psychologic stress situations. *Journal of Nervous and Mental Diseases*, 1952, *115*, 152–162.

Julius, S., & Conway, J. Hemodynamic studies in patients with borderline blood pressure elevation. *Circulation*, 1968, *38*, 282–288.

Kannel, W. B., Gordon, T., & Schwartz, M. J. Systolic versus diastolic blood pressure and risk of coronary heart disease. *American Journal of Cardiology*, 1971, *27*, 335–343.

Kasl, S. V., & Cobb, S. Blood pressure changes in men undergoing job loss: A preliminary report. *Psychosomatic Medicine*, 1970, *32*, 19–38.

Klumbies, G., & Eberhardt, G. Results of autogenic training in the treatment of hypertension. In J. J. Ibor (Ed.), *International Congress Series No. 117*. Amsterdam: Excerpta Medica Foundation, 1966.

Kristt, D. A., & Engel, B. T. Learned control of blood pressure in patients with high blood pressure. *Circulation*, 1975, *51*, 370–378.

Lowenstein, F. W. Blood pressure in relation to age and sex in the tropics and subtropics: A review of the literature and an investigation in two tribes of Brazil Indians. *Lancet*, 1961, *1* (7173), 389–392.

Luthe, W. Autogenic training: Method, research and application in medicine. *American Journal of Psychotherapy*, 1963, *17*, 174–195.

Luthe, W., & Schultz, J. H. (Eds.). *Autogenic therapy, medical applications* (Vol. 2). New York: Grune & Stratton, 1969.

McKegney, F. P., & Williams, R. B. Psychological aspect of hypertension: II. The differential influence of interview variables on blood pressure. *American Journal of Psychiatry*, 1967, *123*, 1539–1543.

Maddocks, I. Possible absence of essential hypertension in two complete Pacific Island populations. *Lancet*, 1961, *7199*, 396–399.

Mahesh Yogi, M. *The Science of being and the art of living*. London: International SRM Publications, 1966.

Marwood, J. F., & Lockett, M. F. Stress induced hypertension in rats. In D. Wheatley (Ed.), *Stress and the heart*. New York: Raven, 1977.

Medoff, H. S., & Bongiovanni, A. M. Blood pressure in rats subjected to audiogenic stimulation. *American Journal of Physiology*, 1945, *143*, 300–305.

Merrill, J. P. Hypertensive vascular disease. In J. V. Harrison, R. D. Adams, I. L. Bennett, W. H. Resnick, G. W. Thorn, & M. M. Wintrobe (Eds.), *Principles of internal medicine*. New York: McGraw-Hill, 1966.

Miasnikov, A. L. The significance of disturbance of higher nervous activity in the pathogenesis of hypertensive disease. In J. H. Cort (Ed.), *Symposium on the pathogenesis of essential hypertension*. Prague: State Medical Publishing House, 1962.

Miller, N. E. Applications of learning and biofeedback to psychiatry and medicine. In A. M. Freedman, H. I. Kaplan, & B. J. Sadock (Eds.), *Comprehensive textbook of psychiatry—II*. Baltimore: Williams & Wilkins, 1975.

Moeller, T. A. *Reduction of arterial blood pressure through relaxation training and correlates of personal-*

ity in hypertensives. Unpublished doctoral dissertation, Nova University, Fort Lauderdale, Florida, 1973.

Mustacchi, P. The interface of the work environment and hypertension. *Medical Clinics of North America,* 1977, *61,* 531–545.

Naditch, M. P. Locus of control, relative discontent and hypertension. *Social Psychiatry,* 1974, *9,* 111–117.

Ostfeld, A., & Lebovits, B. Blood pressure liability: A correlative study. *Journal of Chronic Diseases,* 1960, *12,* 428–439.

Ostfeld, A. M., & D'Atri, D. A. Psychophysiological responses to the urban environment. *International Journal of Psychiatry in Medicine,* 1975, *6,* 15–28.

Patel, C. Twelve-month followup of yoga and biofeedback in the management of hypertension. *Lancet,* 1975, 7898, 62–64. (a)

Patel, C. Yoga and biofeedback in the management of "stress" in hypertensive patients. *Clinical Science and Molecular Medicine,* 1975, *48* (Supplement), 171–174. (b)

Patel, C. Biofeedback-aided relaxation in the management of hypertension. *Biofeedback and Self-Regulation,* 1977, *2,* 1–41.

Patel, C. H. Yoga and biofeedback in the management of hypertension. *Lancet,* 1973, 7837, 1053–1055.

Patel, C. H., & North, W. R. S. Randomized controlled trial of yoga and biofeedback in management of hypertension. *Lancet,* 1975, 7925, 93–95.

Pfeffer, M. A., & Frohlich, E. D. Hemodynamic and myocardial function in young and old normotensive and spontaneously hypertensive rats. *Circulation Research,* 1973, 32–33 (Suppl. 1), 128–135.

Reis, D. Central neural mechanisms governing the criculation with particular reference to the lower brain stem and cerebellum. In A. Zanchetti (Ed.), *Neural and psychological mechanisms in cardiovascular disease.* Milan: Il Ponto, 1972.

Reitan, R. Intellectual and affective changes in essential hypertension. *American Journal of Psychiatry,* 1954, *110,* 817–828.

Reitan, R. A. A research program on the psychological effects of brain lesions in human beings. In N. R. Ellis (Ed.), *International review of research in mental retardation* (Vol. 1). New York: Academic Press, 1966.

Richter-Heinrich, E., & Läuter, J. A psychophysiological test as diagnostic tool with essential hypertensives. *Psychotherapy and Psychomatics,* 1969, *17,* 153–168.

Rushmer, R. F. *Cardiovascular dynamics.* Philadelphia: Saunders, 1970.

Ruskin, A., Beard, O. W., & Schaffer, R. L. "Blast hypertension": Elevated arterial pressures in the victims of the Texas City Disaster. *American Journal of Medicine,* 1948, *4,* 228–236.

Schachter, J. Pain, fear, and anger in hypertensives and normotensives: A psychophysiologic study. *Psychosomatic Medicine,* 1957, *9,* 17–29.

Schultz, J. H., & Luthe, W. *Autogenic therapy* (Vol. 1). New York: Grune & Stratton, 1969.

Schwartz, G. E., & Shapiro, D. Biofeedback and essential hypertension. Current findings and theoretical concerns. *Seminars in Psychiatry,* 1973, *5,* 493–503.

Schwartz, G. E., Shapiro, D., & Tursky, B. Self-control of patterns of human diastolic blood pressure and heart rate through feedback and reward. *Psychophysiology,* 1972, *9,* 270. (Abstract)

Scotch, N. A. Sociological factors in the epidemiology of Zulu hypertension. *American Journal of Public Health,* 1963, *53,* 1205–1213.

Shapiro, A. P. An experimental study of comparative responses of blood pressure to different noxious stimuli. *Journal of Chronic Diseases,* 1961, *13,* 293–311.

Shapiro, A. P., Redmond, D. P., McDonald, R. H., Jr., & Gaylor, M. Relationships of perception, cognition, suggestion and operant conditioning in essential hypertension. *Progress in Brain Research,* 1975, *42,* 299–312.

Shapiro, A. P., Schwartz, G. E., Ferguson, D. C. E., Redmond, D. T., & Weiss, S. M. Behavioral methods in the treatment of hypertension. A review of their clinical status. *Annals of Internal Medicine,* 1977, *86,* 626–636.

Shapiro, D., & Katkin, E. S. Psychophysiological disorders. In A. E. Kazdin, A. S. Bellack, & M. Herson (Eds.), *New perspective in abnormal psychology.* New York: Oxford University Press, 1980.

Shapiro, D., Mainardi, J. A., & Surwit, R. S. Biofeedback and self-regulation in essential hypertension. In G. E. Schwartz & J. Beatty (Eds.), *Biofeedback: Theory and research.* New York: Academic Press, 1977.

Shapiro, D., Schwartz, G. E., & Tursky, B. Control of diastolic blood pressure in man by feedback and reinforcement. *Psychophysiology,* 1972, *9,* 296–304.

Shapiro, D., Tursky, B., Gershon, E., & Stern, M. Effects of feedback and reinforcement on the control of human systolic blood pressure. *Science,* 1969, *163,* 588–590.

Shekelle, R. B., Schoenberger, J. A., & Stamler, J. Correlates of the JAS Type A behavior pattern score. *Journal of Chronic Diseases,* 1976, *29,* 381–394.

Smookler, H. H., Goebel, K. H., Siegel, M. I., & Clarke, D. E. Hypertensive effects of prolonged auditory, visual and motion stimulation. *Federation Proceedings,* 1973, *32,* 2105–2110.

Stahl, S. M., Grim, C. E., Donald, C., & Neikirk, H. J. A model for the social sciences and medicine: The case for hypertension. *Social Science and Medicine,* 1975, *9,* 31–38.

Stokes, G. S., Goldsmith, R. F., Starr, L. M., Gentle, J. L., Mani, M. K., & Stewart, J. H. Plasma renin activity in human hypertension. *Circulation Research,* 1970, *26–27* (Suppl. 2), 207–214.

Stone, R. A., & DeLeo, J. Psychotherapeutic control of hypertension. *New England Journal of Medicine,* 1976, *294,* 80–84.

Surwit, R. S., Shapiro, D., & Good, M. I. A comparison of cardiovascular biofeedback, neuromuscular biofeedback, and meditation in the treatment of borderline essential hypertension. *Journal of Consulting and Clinical Psychology,* 1978, *46,* 252–263.

Taylor, C. B., Farquhar, J. W., Nelson, E., & Agras, S. Relaxation therapy and high blood pressure. *Archives of General Psychiatry,* 1977, *34,* 339–342.

Thacker, E. A. A comparative study of normal and abnormal blood pressures among university students using the cold-pressor test. *American Heart Journal,* 1940, *20,* 89–97.

Tobian, L., Jr. A viewpoint concerning the enigma of hypertension. *American Journal of Medicine,* 1972, *52,* 595–609.

Ueda, H., Kaneko, Y., Takeda, T., Ikeda, K., & Yagi, S. Observations on the mechanism of renin release by hydralazine in hypertensive patients. *Circulation Research,* 1970, *27* (Suppl. 2), 201–206.

Ueda, H., Yasuda, M., Takabatake, Y., Lizuka, M., Lizuka, T., Ihori, M., & Sakamoto, Y. Observations on the mechanism of renin release by catecholamines. *Circulation Research,* 1970, *27* (Suppl. 2), 195–200.

VA Cooperative Study Group on Antihypertensive Agents. Effects of treatment on morbidity in hypertension. i: Results in patients with diastolic blood pressures averaging 115 through 129 mm Hg. *Journal of the American Medical Association,* 1967, *202,* 116–122.

VA Cooperative Study Group on Antihypertensive Agents. Effects of treatment on morbidity in hypertension. ii: Results in patients with diastolic blood pressure averaging 90 through 114 mm Hg. *Journal of the American Medical Association,* 1970, *213,* 1143–1152.

VA Cooperative Study Group on Antihypertensive Agents. Effects of treatment on morbidity in hypertension. iii. Influence of age, diastolic pressure, and prior cardiovascular disease; further analysis of side effects. *Circulation,* 1972, *45,* 991–1004.

Walsh, P., Dale, A., & Anderson, D. E. Comparison of biofeedback pulse wave velocity and progressive relaxation in essential hypertensives. *Perceptual and Motor Skills,* 1977, *44,* 839–843.

Williams, R. B. Heart rate and forearm blood flow feedback in the treatment of a case of severe essential hypertension. *Psychophysiology*, 1975, *12*, 237. (Abstract)

Wolff, H. G., & Wolf, S. The management of hypertensive patients. In E. T. Bell (Ed.), *Hypertension*. Minneapolis: University of Minnesota Press, 1951.

Yeakel, E. H., Shenkin, H. A., Rothballer, A. B., & McCann, S. M. Blood pressure of rats subjected to auditory stimulation. *American Journal of Physiology*, 1948, *155*, 118–127.

7

Raynaud's Disease and Raynaud's Phenomenon

In 1862 Maurice Raynaud published his now famous thesis in which he first described the syndrome today known as Raynaud's disease. Three interrelated phenomena were considered part of his new diagnostic category: local syncope or sudden blanching and numbness of the digits; cyanosis in which the pallor previously observed evolves into a blue color, characteristic of deoxygenated tissue; and reactive hyperemia, characterized by the spread of red oxygenated blood through the upper layers of the epidermis. This last phase is often accompanied by burning and tingling and lasts until the skin returns to its normal pink color. In severe cases, patients experience chronic vasoconstriction or such frequent episodes of cyanosis that gangrene or small nutritive lesions and ulcerations can appear at the distal end of the digits. While vasospasms are usually confined to the digits of the hands and feet, they can occasionally appear on parts of the face as well. Although cold stimulation is the most reliable eliciting stimulus, emotional stress has also been reported to produce these attacks. This is so because the mechanism of peripheral vasoconstriction is essentially mediated by sympathetic tone. This is also why these types of vasospasms are more readily induced by total body cold challenge as opposed to local stimulation. Severe manifestations of this condition are not common, but Lewis (1949) has estimated that it affects approximately 20% of most young people in its mildest forms. Clinical Raynaud's disease is found to occur five times more often in women than in men, the time of onset occurring in the first and second decades of life. When this syndrome results from an identifiable pathological process, it is known as Raynaud's phenomenon (Spittell, 1972).

In order to understand the role of behavior in the etiology, pathogenesis, and treatment of Raynaud's disease, it is important to understand the anatomy of the peripheral vasculature and its regulation by the sympathetic nervous system. With the exception of capillary walls, the walls of all blood vessels are composed of three layers: the itima, the innermost layer; the media, or middle layer, composed mainly of neurally innervated muscular tissue; and the aventitia, or external or sheath, composed mainly of connective tissue. As the large arteries branch out into smaller ones, the ratio of neurally innervated muscular tissue to noninnervated elastic tissue gradually increases to reach a maximum in the arterioles. Thus, the effect of neural control is greatest at the arteriolar level. A similar relationship is found in the venous system. While the veins have a larger lumen and usually a thinner wall, the ratio of smooth muscle fiber to total tissue mass increases as the veins get smaller and smaller down to the level of venules. Unlike arteries, veins also contain a number of valves that prevent retrograde flow in this relatively low-pressure system. Neuromuscular control of blood flow is, thus, most effective at the distal branches of the vascular tree Guglielmi (Note 3).

Two types of vascular structures can be found connecting the arterioles to the venules, thus completing the vascular loop. The capillaries are the most prolific of these structures. Averaging 8 μ in diameter, they have thin walls composed of a single endothelial layer. In general, these vessels lack contractile muscular cells. They serve mainly to supply the tissues with nutrients and oxygen, at the same time removing metabolic waste materials. In addition to the capillaries, there is also a second group of connective vessels, known as the arteriovenous anastomoses. These vessels bypass the capillary network, connecting the arterioles directly to the venules. Unlike capillaries they have a heavy muscular coat that is well supplied with sympathetic fibers. The neural innervation allows enormous amounts of luminal variability, from complete constriction to full dilatation. These structures are most prominent in the skin of the fingers and toes. When the anastomoses are fully dilated, they functionally serve as a shunt, allowing the circulation to bypass the epidermal layers of the peripheral appendages. This peculiar arrangement accounts for the fact that the skin of the extremities, particularly the digits, demonstrates larger circulatory fluctuation than any other area of the body. Wilkins, Doupe, and Newman (1938) have demonstrated that blood flow in the digits can vary up to 600-fold. It is obvious that this enormous range of blood flow in the skin does not serve simple nutritional or metabolic demands alone; it also functions in thermoregulation. The vasculature in the digits can be seen to function much like a radiator in an automobile. This analogy becomes particularly powerful in light of the fact that about 60% of the total body surface is encompassed by the limbs. The opening and closing of the arteriovenous anastomoses can drastically alter the circulation to the skin in response to changes in environmental temperature. Whereas constriction of the anastomoses during exposures to cold reduces peripheral circulation to the minimum needed to maintain metabolic function and hence prevent heat loss, dilatation of the anastomoses provides an efficient heat exchange with the environment mainly through dilated superficial veins. The mechanical function of the anastomoses and dilatation and constriction of the arterioles and venules is primarily governed by the sympathetic nervous system. Coordination and integration of the anatomically mediated vascular responses takes place at the medullary, diencephalic, and cortical levels. The hypothalamus as well as areas in the medulla have been shown to be crucial in this process (see Bard, 1963; Folkow, 1955, 1956 for review). The powerful effect of this central thermoregulatory mechanism was demonstrated by Rapaport, Fetcher, and Hall (1948). They showed that when the body was sufficiently heated, bare hands and feet would remain warm and vasodilated even when exposed to ambient temperatures as low as $-34°C$. Therefore, although the effect of bradykinen, the axon reflex, and other local vasoregulatory mechanisms are important in thermoregulation, the central effect of the sympathetic nervous system on the vasculature in its attempt to maintain thermoregulation is paramount (Burton & Edholm, 1954).

While there is substantial agreement about the existence of one or more active vasodilatory mechanisms in the proximal portions of the limbs, vascular control of the peripheral vessels of the digits is thought to be purely a result of sympathetically mediated vasconstriction. More specifically, vasoconstriction of the arterioles and venules as well as anastomoses is mediated by alpha-adrenergic sympathetic receptors. Postganglionic axons are adrenergic, unmyelinated C-fibers that are continuously active. This activity maintains vasomotor tone, which in part helps maintain blood pressure. By firing at a rate of one or two times per second, these peripheral sympathetic nerves maintain a constant state of contraction in the peripheral vascular tree. The level of contraction is modulated by an increase or decrease in sympathetic nervous system activity. Increasing sympathetic activity will provide a greater amount of vasoconstriction, while vasodilatation can be brought about by decreases in sympathetic activity. Although this simple control mechanism is found in most sympathetically innervated vessels, it is most prominent in the cutaneous and distal portions of the limbs, in particular the hands and feet, where the arteriovenous anastomoses are found.

Since the vasoconstrictive mechanism of the arterioles, venules, and anastomoses is thought to be alpha-adrenergic, the vascular smooth muscle of these structures is responsive to humoral as well as direct neural stimulation. Central activation of the sympathetic nervous system produces both direct sympathetic stimulation through the postganglionic fibers as well as humoral stimulation through release of epinephrine by the adrenal medulla. Cortisol, secreted by the adrenal cortex, can potentiate these effects by sensitizing alpha-receptors to these catecholamines (Mendowitz, Gitlow, & Naftchi, 1958). The importance of these humoral mechanisms in the control of vasoconstriction is underscored by the fact that peripheral vasoconstriction can still occur following sympathectomies.

Although the primary function of this sympathetically mediated vasoconstrictor system is thermoregulatory, the system is exquisitely responsive to higher cortical activity. In fact, any stimulus to which an animal attends can produce a vasoconstrictive response in these peripheral vessels. Sokolow(1963) describes this reaction as part of the "orienting reflex," which occurs in response to all stimuli that have "signal value" to the organism. That the central nervous system (CNS) can affect this otherwise "reflexive" response system is crucial to the understanding of how behavior interacts with peripheral vascular disease.

PATHOPHYSIOLOGY OF RAYNAUD'S DISEASE

The pathophysiology of Raynaud's disease is not completely understood. While Raynaud himself attributed the malady to sympathetic overreactivity, Lewis (1949) maintained that the problem resulted from a local fault in the peripheral digital vessels. He collected evidence showing that changes in environmental temperature could have specific effects on the part of the digits stimulated by cold. Lewis did not believe that the patients he examined who were suffering from Raynaud's disease were abnormally "nervous." This led him to downplay the contribution of emotional and CNS activity upon the manifestations of this disorder.

Mittelmann and Wolff (1939) demonstrated that emotional stress could reduce the digital blood flow as measured by skin temperature in both normals and Raynaud's patients. In Raynaud's patients, however, these changes in temperature were accompanied by the blanching–cyanotic–edemic color change and pain typical of the vasospastic disorder. They reported that temperature changes were not in and of themselves sufficient cause for the vasospasm. Rather, the attacks seemed to occur most reliably when emotional stress and low environmental temperature interacted. In addition, they failed to find emotional stimuli effective in producing this reaction after sympathectomy. Graham (1955) was also able to demonstrate the vasoconstrictive effects of disturbing interviews on the skin temperature of both patients with Raynaud's disease as well as normal subjects. In addition, he was able to isolate hostility and anxiety as the emotions most often responsible for this reaction. In a subsequent study, Graham, Stern, and Winokur (1958) demonstrated that, by suggesting these emotions to normal subjects under hypnosis, vasoconstriction in the digits could be produced.

Although this evidence strongly implies that emotional stimuli are at least a contributing factor in the elicitation of Raynaud's disease, the local-fault hypothesis of Lewis cannot be immediately ruled out. Mendowitz and Naftchi

(1959) have suggested that Raynaud's disease might be dichotomized into two separate disorders: one in which the vasculature is normal and vasomotor tone is heightened by sympathetic overreactivity and another in which normal vasomotor tone produces an overreaction in pathological local vasculature.

Much of the dispute as to the etiology of Raynaud's disease is probably attributable to diagnostic confusion. Allen and Brown (1932) produced one of the first attempts to improve on the nosological categories established by Maurice Raynaud. They suggested the following criteria for the diagnosis of true idiopathic Raynaud's disease: (*a*) intermittent attacks of discoloration of the extremities, (*b*) absence of evidence of organic arterial occlusion, (*c*) symmetrical or bilateral distribution, (*d*) trophic changes, when present, limited to skin and never consisting of gross gangrene, (*e*) disease present for at least 2 years, and (*f*) no evidence of any other disease that could produce the symptoms secondarily. More recently Holling (1972) described the idiopathic condition as "spasmodic contraction of the arteries and small arteries of the fingers leading to the slowing or cessation of the blood flow. It is provoked by exposure to cold and sometimes by emotion. The affected fingers are pallid or cyanosed and cold and red and painful during the recovery phase [p. 140]." Furthermore, he notes that there should be no signs of underlying circulatory pathology, the symptoms should be intermittent with a normal pulse appearing when the body is warmed by an external heat source. Gifford and Hines (1957) and DeTakats and Fowler (1962) cautioned that a period of at least 16 years may separate the first evidence of vasospasm from the appearance of scleroderma. Thus, the 2-year requirement proposed by Allen and Brown is probably insufficient to rule out other pathology. Although some rheumatologists argue that all Raynaud's disease is a precursor to some latent rheumatological condition, we have seen many cases of people with a 40-year history of symptoms that have not been progressive. Nonetheless, Porter and colleagues (Porter, Bardana, Baur, Wesche, Andrasch, & Rosch, 1976), in reviewing a large series of cases in which "Raynaud's-like" vasospasms were the first and only presenting symptom, found that nearly 80% could be shown to have some autoimmune or other dysfunction.

Surwit and colleagues (Surwit, Allen, Kuhn, Gilgor, Duvic, Schandberg, & Williams, 1981) have suggested that idiopathic Raynaud's disease is associated with a different neuroendocrine response to cold than Raynaud's phenomenon. Whereas the neuroendocrine response to cold of patients with Raynaud's phenomenon is essentially normal, patients with idiopathic Raynaud's disease show significantly lower levels of plasma norepinephrine in response to cold in the presence of high cortisol levels. Thus, idiopathic Raynaud's disease appears to result from more than an excess of sympathetic nervous system activity.

Raynaud's phenomenon can be caused by scleroderma and other collagen disorders in which the vasculature is attacked by excessive amounts of collagen deposits. Lupus erythematosis also produces symptoms of Raynaud's phenomenon, which in this case can be attributed to the vascular inflammation characteristic of this disease. In both cases, the symptoms of Raynaud's phenomenon are much more severe than those of idiopathic Raynaud's disease. Nutritive lesions and gangrenous ulcers tend to be prominent, often necessitating amputation of the distal parts of the digits. Raynaud's-like phenomena are also associated with thromboangitis obliterans, arteriosclerosis obliterans, obstruction due to emboli or thromboses, intoxication from heavy metals, rheumatoid arthritis, dermatomyocytis, angiocarotoma corpus diffusum, proximal hemoglobinuria, cryoglobulemia, primary hypertension, myxedema, and such occupational-trauma-related disorders as pneumatic hammer disease, occupational occlusive arterial disease, vasospastic phenomenon of typists and pianists, denervation trauma, shoulder girdle compression syndrome, carpal tunnel syndrome, and other neurological diseases. While there is some indication that Raynaud's phenomenon secondary to scleroderma or lupus erythematosis may be relieved symptomatically by behavioral intervention, these other causes of peripheral vascular disease must be primarily addressed medically.

MEDICAL TREATMENT OF RAYNAUD'S DISEASE

Until recently, medical treatment of Raynaud's disease was largely prophylactic. Patients were characteristically instructed to dress warmly, to avoid exposure to cold, and, if their condition was severe, to move to a warmer climate (Pratt, 1949). Surgical treatment via sympathectomy, while effective in reducing vasospasms in the lower extremities, has yielded unreliable results in the upper extremities (Spittell, 1972) and leaves permanent side effects (Patton, 1965). Medical therapy with agents that suppress sympathetic vasomotor activity is the most common form of treatment. Abboud, Eckstein, Lawrence, and Hoak (1967), Kontos and Wasserman (1969), and Romeo, Whalen, and Tindall (1970) have shown that reserpine can decrease both the frequency and severity of vasospastic attacks in patients with Raynaud's disease. Kontos and Wasserman also reported that equally good results could be obtained by administration of guanethadine and therefore concluded that therapeutic benefit resulted from a catecholamine-depleting effect and consequent decrease in adrenergic activity. Varadi and Lawrence (1969) used methyldopa to prevent vasospastic attacks in 42 patients who were exposed to experimental cold. These results also support the notion that decreasing adrenergic activity is important in producing clinical improvement. Finally, Spittell (1972) reported that doses of 25–50 mg of tolazoline (a vasodilator with alpha-adrenergic blocking potential) three to four times a day is helpful in the management of mild Raynaud's disease. But, as the severity of the disease increases, the side effects produced by the medication begin to outweigh the therapeutic benefit. The problem of side effects is extremely important in any of the aforementioned treatments. Reserpine, even given in small doses, can have a profound effect on the CNS and produces severe depression and even suicidal behavior, increased appetite, weight gain, as well as gastrointestinal complications (Nickerson, 1970). Methyldopa can also provoke depression and gastrointestinal complications as well as lactation, extrapyramidal signs, and liver damage (Nickerson, 1970). Tolazoline can cause tachycardia, cardiac arrhythmias, anginal pain, and gastrointestinal disturbance and may even be a precipitating factor in myocardial infarction (Nickerson, 1970). In summary, while these and other drugs may produce some symptomatic relief of Raynaud's disease, administration of these substances often cause intolerable side effects, especially when symptom severity demands vigorous treatment. More importantly, because most of these agents tend to work by reducing alpha-adrenergic activity, either locally or centrally, it is plausible that a behavioral intervention aimed at producing a central decrease in sympathetic activity could have equal therapeutic benefit.

BEHAVIORAL TREATMENT OF RAYNAUD'S DISEASE AND PHENOMENON

Recently there has been a great deal of interest in the possibility that patients suffering from vasospastic symptoms of Raynaud's disease could benefit from learning control of peripheral vasodilatation. Interest in this area initially grew from the successful reports of learned control of peripheral blood flow in normals, which we reviewed earlier (see Chapter 4). A number of clinical researchers attempted to extend the methods developed in these initial laboratory studies to application with patients suffering from Raynaud's disease and phenomenon. In this section we will review the published studies in this area. Although most of these studies deal with the application of biofeedback to Raynaud's disease, there are also a number of investigations that attempt to assess the efficacy of other behavioral techniques in dealing with Raynaud's disease and phenomenon.

Biofeedback

In the first study in which patients suffering from Raynaud's disease were trained to increase peripheral blood flow, two patients suffering from primary

Raynaud's disease were provided with biofeedback of blood volume changes as recorded by a photoplethysmograph (Shapiro & Schwartz, 1972). Feedback of blood volume changes occurring in the finger was provided to one patient, while the other patient was provided with feedback of blood volume changes recorded from the toes. The treatment was moderately successful for one patient, who reported a reduction in the severity of Raynaud's symptoms. The treatment was unsuccessful in the other patient. This study is unique in that it is the only published study in which feedback of blood volume changes has been used to facilitate learned control of peripheral blood flow.

Surwit (1973) was the first to report the systematic use of skin temperature biofeedback in the treatment of a case of Raynaud's disease. The patient in this study was a 21-year-old female who reported vasospasms occurring in both hands and feet. The patient previously had bilateral cervical and lumbar sympathectomies. The cervical sympathectomy was unsuccessful and, because the woman lived in a very cold climate (Montreal, Canada), she underwent a considerable number of vasospasms each year. This patient was subjected to a very intensive course of behavioral training. She was initially trained in autogenic and progressive relaxation techniques and then provided with a series of 52 laboratory biofeedback sessions spaced over a 9-month period. During training, feedback was provided by a computer cathode-ray tube (CRT) that displayed a cumulative record of skin temperature while an audible bell underscored each .1°C increase in skin temperature. Over 4 months of training, the patient's basal hand temperature rose from 23.3°C to 26.6°C, and a concomitant decrease in the frequency of Raynaud's attacks was reported. When the patient was contacted for a 9-year follow-up, she indicated that she continues to practice voluntary control and claimed a continued maintenance of therapeutic effect.

The use of hypnosis and biofeedback in the treatment of Raynaud's disease was reported by Jacobson, Hackett, Surman, and Silverberg (1973). In this case, the patient showed very little improvement during the hypnosis portion of training. However, when the patient was provided with temperature biofeedback designed to teach him to increase finger temperature relative to forehead temperature, a marked reduction in the frequency of Raynaud's attacks occurred. These gains were maintained at 8-month follow-up. As contrasted with the earlier work of Surwit (1973), this study placed less emphasis on laboratory training and much more emphasis on the importance of the patient's practice with self-control techniques at home. No follow-up is reported.

Blanchard and Haynes (1975) have conducted the most systematic and controlled single-case study published to date. In this study, changes in skin temperature and the frequency of Raynaud's attacks were evaluated under three conditions: (a) no-treatment baseline, (b) self-control technique in which the patient was asked to try to increase her hand temperature any way she could, and (c) biofeedback training to increase hand relative to forehead temperature. The results provided strong support for the utility of temperature biofeedback. During the biofeedback sessions, the patient showed an ability to increase her hand temperature an average of 3.4°F, whereas no consistent changes in temperature were noted under any of the other conditions. The authors also reported a gradual increase in basal finger temperature from 79°F to 91.1°F. Reductions in the frequency of vasospasms were achieved concurrent with temperature biofeedback training. Follow-up evaluations at 2 and 4 months revealed maintenance of treatment gains. Although control over skin temperature had deteriorated by 7 months posttreatment, acquisition of learned control was reinstated after five additional training sessions. No long-term follow-up is available.

The most recent and also one of the most poorly controlled single-case studies was reported by Sunderman and Delk (1978). In this study, a 40-year-old patient with a 15-year history of Raynaud's disease was provided with temperature biofeedback to teach her to increase hand temperature. During biofeedback sessions, the patient was encouraged to use whatever technique would provide temperature increases. She arrived at a strategy of subvocally quoting biblical scriptures and, by the end of training, actually brought the Bible to the sessions. The patient had a long course of treatment—three sessions a week for 13 months. In addition to the biofeedback and subvocal biblical quoting, the patient was also on medication. Although the authors reported that this patient showed gradual temperature changes over the course of treatment, the unorthodox combination of treatment procedures makes it very difficult to determine what elements were responsible for the change.

Findings similar to these just reviewed have been reported in numerous unpublished case studies. Looking at these studies in the best light, one can say that they suggest that certain patients suffering from Raynaud's disease can learn control over skin temperature, show a reduction in the frequency of attacks, and maintain these changes over long periods. However, if one examines these studies from a more critical viewpoint, a number of problems are evident. Most important is external validity; that is, how would the results achieved with any of these individual patients generalize to a larger population of patients?

The results of these case studies seem to suggest that temperature biofeedback training may be helpful in the treatment of Raynaud's disease. However, the primary source of outcome data in all these studies is self-report. Self-report is a notoriously inaccurate and biased method of evaluating treatment (Keefe, Kopel, & Gordon, 1978), which can be influenced strongly by the demand characteristics of the situation. In an effort to provide a more stringent measure of learned control of peripheral vasodilatation, a number of researchers have suggested that one examine the ability of the patients to maintain hard temperature under cold ambient stress. Taub (1977) described using such a procedure with Raynaud's patients. In this study, patients who had been trained in temperature self-control were fitted with a "cold suit" and instructed to attempt to maintain hand temperature as the temperature in the suit varied. This suit was designed in such a way that cold water of specified temperatures could be rapidly circulated so that the patient's whole body could be stressed. Taub has reported on the results achieved with only one patient so far. This patient was able to actually increase hand temperature from 88°F to 89.5°F while the temperature of the cold suit was decreased from 80°F to 60°F. Unfortunately, no data are provided on the clinical changes observed in this patient.

In each of the case studies presented, the number of subjects was small and no statistical treatment of the data was presented. Because only cases in which such treatment techniques are successful are published, the number of failures goes unreported. Without a no-treatment or other appropriate control group, the therapeutic gains reported cannot be honestly attributed to biofeedback. Finally, in each study multiple treatment techniques were used. When treatment effects are analyzed over such a long period, the possibility of carry-over effects from one treatment to another is strong. Although patients may show changes during temperature biofeedback sessions, these changes may be mediated by a cognitive strategy previously taught to the patient, for example, self-hypnosis or autogenic training. It seems fair to conclude, however, that these studies suggest that behavioral techniques such as biofeedback may have an important role to play in the management of patients with Raynaud's symptoms. Recently, controlled group outcome studies have attempted to address more systematically the potential contribution particular behavioral techniques may provide.

Relaxation and Other Techniques

A series of controlled studies investigating the behavioral treatment of Raynaud's disease have been conducted. These studies have attempted to identify the relative contribution of particular behavioral techniques in facilitating self-control of skin temperature and reducing Raynaud's attacks. In the first study of the series (Surwit, Pilon, & Fenton, 1978), two major questions were addressed. What contribution did biofeedback make to a course of autogenic training in the control of hand temperature? And, does autogenic or biofeedback training need to be performed under laboratory conditions in order for patients to benefit?

Thirty female patients diagnosed as suffering from idiopathic Raynaud's disease were trained to control their digital skin temperature using either autogenic training or a combination of autogenic training and skin temperature feedback. Training was conducted either in a laboratory or in three group sessions supplemented by extensive home practice. All subjects were exposed to an initial cold stress procedure in which they were seated in an experimental chamber while the ambient temperature was slowly dropped from 26°C to 17°C over 72 min. Skin temperature, heart rate, and pulse amplitudes were monitored during the temperature change. This procedure was given to half the subjects immediately before and immediately following a 4-week training sequence. The remaining half of the sample was exposed to an additional cold stress challenge prior to treatment as a control for possible habituation effects. The results of this study are illustrated in Figure 7.1. All subjects, regardless of which condition they were trained in, showed a significant improvement in their ability to maintain digital skin temperature relative both to their initial cold stress as well as to the second cold stress given to the half of the sample not immediately treated. Patients who served as a no-treatment control not only failed to show improvement during the second test but actually deteriorated in performance. In addition to this objective finding, all treated patients reported significant reductions in the frequency of vasospastic attacks over the 4-week treatment period. No additional benefits could be observed for those subjects receiving skin temperature biofeedback or for those subjects whose training was conducted in the laboratory (see Figure 7.2).

The second study of this series (Keefe, Surwit, & Pilon, 1980) served as a partial replication as well as an extension of the study just described. This

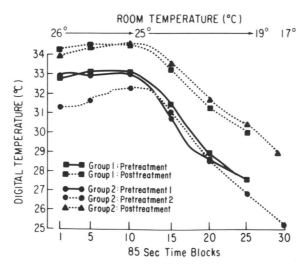

FIGURE 7.1. Mean digital temperature during pre- and posttreatment stress tests. Recording of skin temperature begun after a 10-min stabilization period. [From R. S. Surwit, R. N. Pilon, & C. H. Fenton. Behavioral treatment of Raynaud's disease. *Journal of Behavioral Medicine*, 1978, *1*, 329.]

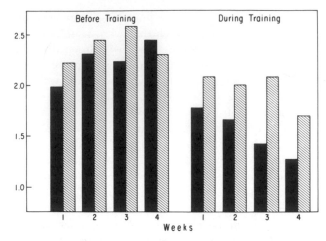

FIGURE 7.2. Mean number and intensity of attacks per day reported by all subjects during the 4 weeks immediately preceding training and the 4 weeks of training. The reduction in the number of attacks across weeks of treatment was significant. [From R. S. Surwit, R. N. Pilon, & C. H. Fenton. Behavioral treatment of Raynaud's disease. *Journal of Behavioral Medicine,* 1978, *1,* 331. Solid bars indicate mean number of attacks per day. Ruled bars indicate mean intensity of attacks per day (on a 1–5 scale).]

second study attempted to provide a more rigorous test of home biofeedback training by having patients on home practice regimens use more sophisticated and sensitive temperature feedback equipment than had been used in the prior study. This study also compared the efficacy of autogenic training (which focuses specifically upon sensations of warmth and heaviness in the hands) to general relaxation training (which focuses upon reducing muscular tension generally throughout the body). In addition, this study used four laboratory cold stress challenges like those described in the previous study given at week 1 of a 4-week baseline and during weeks 1, 3, and 5 of training. Twenty-one patients were randomly assigned to one of three treatment conditions. The first group received progressive muscle relaxation and home practice instructions; the second group received autogenic training and home practice instructions; while the third group received autogenic training and skin temperature feedback with autogenic instructions and portable skin temperature feedback equipment. The results confirmed those of the initial study in that all patients improved regardless of treatment (see Figure 7.3). Data gathered from the cold stress procedures indicated that subjects improved gradually and significantly over the four cold stress challenges. This improvement was not felt to be due to habituation since the initial study had indicated that patients deteriorated in performance without training. The gradual improvement of the response to the cold stress procedure suggests that some learning process was taking place. As previously

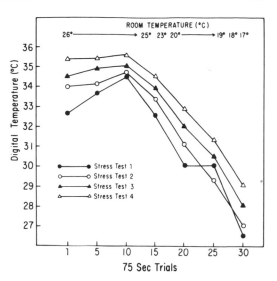

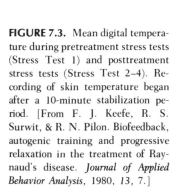

FIGURE 7.3. Mean digital temperature during pretreatment stress tests (Stress Test 1) and posttreatment stress tests (Stress Test 2–4). Recording of skin temperature began after a 10-minute stabilization period. [From F. J. Keefe, R. S. Surwit, & R. N. Pilon. Biofeedback, autogenic training and progressive relaxation in the treatment of Raynaud's disease. *Journal of Applied Behavior Analysis*, 1980, *13*, 7.]

reported, all treated patients also experienced an approximate 40% reduction in the frequency of vasospastic attacks. This reduction in symptoms was obtained at the same time as a significant drop in ambient outdoor temperature was occurring.

Another group of investigators obtained similar results. Jacobson, Manschreck, and Silverberg (1979) gave 12 patients suffering from idiopathic Raynaud's disease 12 sessions of muscle relaxation training over a 6-week period. Half of the patients were also given auditory and visual skin temperature feedback during the training sessions. Skin temperature during training as well as patients' self-reports of improvement were recorded. Both groups showed significant increases in skin temperature during training, with larger skin temperature increases shown by the group not receiving feedback. All subjects rated themselves moderately to markedly improved at 1 month with 7 subjects continuing to report improvement at 2 years. No data were collected on objective hand temperature changes at follow-up.

In the final study (Keefe, Surwit, & Pilon, 1979), the maintenance of treatment gains was evaluated. Nineteen patients who had undergone behavioral training in the initial study (Surwit *et al.*, 1978) were asked to keep a daily log of frequency and severity of vasospastic attacks and to fill in a follow-up questionnaire dealing with their satisfaction with various elements in the treatment regimen. One year after initial treatment, these patients were given an additional cold stress challenge. Thus, as before, both objective and subjective indexes of symptom improvement were obtained. The results of the study are fascinating in that they appear on the surface to be contradictory. One year

posttreatment, patients reported an average of 1.2 vasospasms per day, compared to 1.3 attacks per day immediately following treatment 1 year earlier.
However, the ability of patients to maintain digital temperature in the face of
cold stress had significantly deteriorated and was virtually identical to their
initial treatment performance (see Figures 7.4 and 7.5). The contradiction
implied by these two sets of data can be explained by examining data from the
follow-up questionnaire administered to all patients. Most patients had stopped
practicing the behavioral techniques during the spring months following their
initial training. These patients had not returned to levels of practice comparable to those they were engaged in during the initial treatment. Thus, while
response to performance during cold stress was seen as related to practice, the
patient's subjective reports of improvement seem to be under the control of other
variables.

   Two other explanations can be offered to explain the discrepancy between
subjects continuing to report fewer vasospastic attacks despite a deterioration of
their ability to tolerate the cold stress challenge. First, it is possible that
subjects were simply trying to please the investigators by reporting fewer vasospastic attacks. It is well known that different variables control verbal and
nonverbal behavior (Keefe, Kopel, & Gordon, 1978). However, it is also possible that subjects did retain some control of their ability to voluntarily

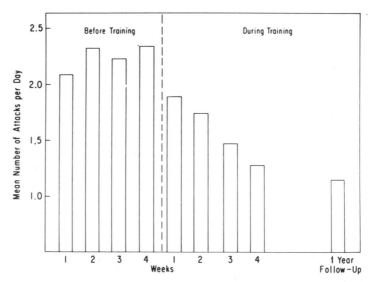

FIGURE 7.4. Mean frequency of vasospastic attacks recorded during the 4 weeks before training,
the 4 weeks posttraining, and a 1-week 1-year follow-up. [From F. J. Keefe, R. S. Surwit, & R. N.
Pilon. A one year follow-up of Raynaud's patients treated with behavioral therapy techniques.
Journal of Behavioral Medicine, 1979, 2, 389.]

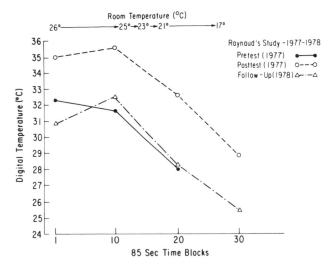

FIGURE 7.5. Mean digital temperature (°C) during cold stress tests conducted pretreatment, posttreatment, and at a 1-year follow-up. [From F. J. Keefe, R. S. Surwit, & R. N. Pilon. A one year follow-up of Raynaud's patients treated with behavioral therapy techniques. *Journal of Behavioral Medicine*, 1979, 2, 388.]

vasodilate—enough to prevent vasospasms but not enough to meet the challenge of the cold stress test. Mittelmann and Wolff (1939) demonstrated that a drop in digital temperature alone is not sufficient to bring on a vasospasm. Low digital temperature is a precursor to vasospasm, they noted, only if the subject is autonomically aroused.

A study by Surwit, Bradner, Fenton, and Pilon (1979) sheds some light on which behavioral variables may be important in predicting the response of patients to a behavioral program designed to treat Raynaud's disease. These investigators found that subjects' improvements, as measured by increased skin temperature during the cold stress test, could be predicted by subjects' responses to a simple paper-and-pencil test. Thirty subjects, trained in voluntary vasomotor control with skin temperature feedback and autogenic training, were given the Psychological Screening Inventory (Lanyon, 1973). Those subjects scoring high in the alienation scale of this inventory were found to show no improvement in skin temperature in response to cold stress, whereas those subjects with low scores showed a net increase of 4.5°C after training. According to Lanyon (1973), high scores on the alienation scale are associated with high scores on those scales on the Minnesota Multiphasic Personality Inventory related to serious psychopathology (schizophrenia, infrequency, paranoia, hypomania). People with high scores on this scale perceive themselves as not responsible for or in control of their own lives. Thus, this scale appears sensitive to a feeling of self-control, which seems important for success in treatments based on exercise of self-control.

Several investigators have reported on the use of biofeedback and other behavioral techniques in treating Raynaud's phenomenon secondary to scleroderma. May and Weber (Note 1) were the first to report on the use of skin temperature feedback to treat the digital vasospasms that result from this disorder. Five patients with Raynaud's phenomenon, three of whom had been diagnosed as suffering from scleroderma, were given skin temperature biofeedback. All patients, including those suffering from scleroderma, were able to raise skin temperature in the laboratory, and all reported decreased frequency of vasospasms. Keefe, Surwit, and Pilon (in press) trained one patient suffering from Raynaud's phenomenon secondary to mixed connective tissue disease using the autogenic and biofeedback techniques described by Surwit *et al.* (1978). In addition to decreased self-reports of vasospasms, this patient showed increased resistance to multiple cold stress procedures over a 7-month training period. By the end of this period, the patient was able to demonstrate a 7°C increase in digital temperature compared to baseline. Finally, Freedman, Ianni, Hale, and Lynn (1979) trained two patients with diagnosed scleroderma and Raynaud's phenomenon to control skin temperature using temperature feedback alone. Both patients received 12 biweekly training sessions. The patients were able to show voluntary vasodilatation with feedback accompanied by a decrease in reported vasospasms. The skin temperature of the two patients was monitored in the field by telemetry. An increase in skin temperature over pretraining levels was observed in a variety of conditions. Freedman (Note 2) has added four more patients to the same protocol, with similar positive results.

CONCLUSION

The foregoing review allows us to draw the following conclusions about the utility of biofeedback and self-control procedures in the treatment of Raynaud's disease. First, it appears that biofeedback, especially when used with autogenic training or hypnosis, provides a reliable behavioral treatment for Raynaud's disease. Investigators have described both subjective reductions of symptomatology as well as objective indexes of increased blood flow under conditions of cold stress subsequent to training. Typically, patients report up to 50% reduction in symptom frequency following training, with the increase of resting digital temperature approximately 3–4°C. These results are impressive and parallel the best clinical effects of many medical as well as surgical interventions. Although there are many fewer data on the use of these techniques in treating Raynaud's phenomenon, the data that do exist suggest that vasospasms secondary to collagen-vascular disease are behaviorally treatable as well.

However, when we attempt to separate biofeedback from a general package of behavioral interventions, the peculiar contribution of biofeedback to therapy becomes difficult to discern. In the three controlled group outcome studies just reviewed, there is typically no difference in efficacy between relaxation techniques or relaxation techniques supplemented with biofeedback. Another study, however, does tend to point out a difference in therapeutic efficacy between biofeedback-assisted and non-biofeedback-assisted relaxation procedures. Surwit and Fenton (1980) compared the performance of subjects during autogenic training both with and without skin temperature feedback. Eight subjects received eight sessions of feedback-assisted autogenic instructions, while eight subjects received eight sessions of autogenic training alone. Typically, all subjects showed a .3°C rise from baseline during the 5-min interval when they were given auditory autogenic instructions. Following the playing of the tapes, subjects were asked to recite the autogenic phrases to themselves over a 72-min period. However, those subjects receiving skin temperature feedback were able to maintain higher levels of digital temperature throughout the course of the session. Thus, while autogenic instructions or suggestion were seen as responsible for initial changes in vasomotor tone, feedback did seem to be of some help in allowing subjects to maintain these changes.

REFERENCE NOTES

1. May, D. S., & Weber, C. A. Temperature feedback training for symptom reduction in primary and secondary Raynaud's disease. Unpublished manuscript, 1976.
2. Freedman, R. Personal communication, April 1980.
3. Guglielmi, R. S. Raynaud's disease: Neurogenic or local fault? A critical review of the evidence. Unpublished manuscript, 1976.

REFERENCES

Abboud, F. M., Eckstein, J. W., Lawrence, M. S., & Hoak, J. C. Preliminary observations on the use of intra-arterial reserpine in Raynaud's phenomenon. *Circulation*, 1967, 36 (no. 4, Suppl. II), II–49. (Abstract)

Allen, E. V., & Brown, G. E. Raynaud's disease: A critical review of the minimal requisite for diagnosis. *American Journal of Medical Sciences*, 1932, 183, 187–200.

Bard, P. Central nervous control of vascular flow. In J. L. Orbison & D. E. Smith (Eds.), *The peripheral blood vessels*. Baltimore: Williams & Wilkins, 1963.

Blanchard, E. B., & Haynes, M. R. Biofeedback treatment of a case of Raynaud's disease. *Journal of Behavior Therapy and Experimental Psychiatry*, 1975, 6, 230–234.

Burton, A. C., & Edholm, O. G. *Man in a cold environment; Physiological and pathological effects of exposure to low temperatures.* Baltimore: Williams & Wilkins, 1954.

DeTakats, G., & Fowler, E. F. Raynaud's phenomenon. *Journal of the American Medical Association,* 1962, *179,* 1–8.

Folkow, B. Nervous control of the blood vessels. *Physiological Review,* 1955, *35,* 629–663.

Folkow, B. The nervous control of the blood vessels. In R. J. S. McDowell (Ed.), *The control of the circulation of the blood* (Vol. 2). London: Dawson, 1956.

Freedman, R., Ianni, P., Hale, P., & Lynn, S. Treatment of Raynaud's phenomenon with biofeedback and cold desensitization. *Psychophysiology,* 1979, *16,* 182. (Abstract)

Gifford, R. W., Jr., & Hines, E. A., Jr. Raynaud's disease among women and girls. *Circulation,* 1957, *16,* 1012–1021.

Graham, D. T. Cutaneous vascular reactions in Raynaud's disease and in states of hostility, anxiety, and depression. *Psychosomatic Medicine,* 1955, *17,* 200–207.

Graham, D. T., Stern, J. A., & Winokur, C. Experimental investigation of the specficity of attitude hypothesis in psychosomatic disease. *Psychosomatic Medicine,* 1958, *20,* 446–457.

Holling, H. E. *Peripheral vascular diseases: Diagnosis and management.* Philadelphia: Lippincott, 1972.

Jacobson, A. M., Hackett, T. P., Surman, O. S., & Silverberg, E. L. Raynaud's phenomenon: Treatment with hypnotic and operant technique. *Journal of the American Medical Association,* 1973, *225,* 739–740.

Jacobson, A. M., Manschreck, T. C., & Silverberg, E. Behavioral treatment for Raynaud's Disease: A comparative study with long-term follow-up. *American Journal of Psychiatry,* 1979, *136,* 844–846.

Keefe, F. J., Kopel, S., & Gordon, S. *A practical guide to behavioral assessment.* New York: Springer, 1978.

Keefe, F. J., Surwit, R. S., & Pilon, R. N. Collagen vascular disease: Can behavior therapy help? *Behavior Therapy and Experimental Psychiatry,* in press.

Keefe, F. J., Surwit, R. S., & Pilon, R. N. A one-year follow-up of Raynaud's patients treated with behavioral therapy techniques. *Journal of Behavioral Medicine,* 1979, *2,* 385–391.

Keefe, F. J., Surwit, R. S., & Pilon, R. N. Biofeedback, autogenic training and progressive relaxation in the treatment of Raynaud's disease. *Journal of Applied Behavior Analysis,* 1980, *13,* 3–11.

Kontos, H. A., & Wasserman, A. J. Effects of Reserpine in Raynaud's phenomenon. *Circulation,* 1969, *39,* 259–266.

Lanyon, R. I. *Psychological screening inventory: Manual.* Goshen, N.Y.: Research Psychologists' Press, 1973.

Lewis, T. *Vascular disorders of the limbs: Described for practitioners and students.* London: Macmillan, 1949.

Mendlowitz, M., & Naftchi, N. The digital circulation in Raynaud's disease. *American Journal of Cardiology,* 1959, *4,* 580–584.

Mendowitz, M., Gitlow, S., & Naftchi, N. Work of digital vasoconstriction produced by infused norepinephrine in Cushing's Syndrome. *Journal of Applied Physiology,* 1958, *13,* 252–256.

Mittelmann, B., & Wolff, H. G. Affective states and skin temperature: Experimental study of subjects with "cold hands" and Raynaud's syndrome. *Psychosomatic Medicine,* 1939, *1,* 271–292.

Nickerson, M. Vasodilator drugs. In L. S. Goodman & A. Gilman (Eds.), *The pharmacological basis of therapeutics.* New York: Macmillan, 1970.

Patton, H. D. The autonomic nervous system. In T. C. Ruch, H. D. Patton, J. W. Woodbury, & A. L. Towe (Eds.), *Neurophysiology.* Philadelphia: Saunders, 1965.

Porter, J. M., Bardana, E. J., Baur, G. M., Wesche, D. H., Andrasch, R. H., & Rosch, J. The clinical significance of Raynaud's Syndrome. *Surgery,* 1976, *80,* 756–764.

Pratt, G. H. *Surgical management of vascular disease.* Philadelphia: Lea & Febiger, 1949.

Rapaport, S. I., Fetcher, E. S., & Hall, J. F. Physiological protection of the extremities from severe cold. *Federation Proceedings,* 1948, *7,* 99. (Abstract)

Raynaud, M. *De l'asphyxie locale et de la gangrène symétrique des extrémités.* Paris: Rignoux, 1862.

Romeo, S. G., Whalen, R. E., & Tindall, J. P. Intra-arterial administration of reserpine. Its use in patients with Raynaud's disease or Raynaud's phenomenon. *Archives of Internal Medicine,* 1970, *125,* 825–829.

Shapiro, D., & Schwartz, G. E. Biofeedback and visceral learning: Clinical applications. *Seminars in Psychiatry,* 1972, *4,* 171–184.

Sokolow, Y. N. *Perception and the conditioned reflex,* London: Pergamon, 1963.

Spittell, J. A., Jr. Raynaud's phenomenon and allied vasospastic conditions. In J. F. Fairbairn, J. C. Juergens, & A. Spittell (Eds.), *Allen-Barker-Hines peripheral vascular diseases* (4th ed.). Philadelphia: Saunders, 1972.

Sunderman, R. H., & Delk, J. L, Treatment of Raynaud's disease with temperature biofeedback. *Southern Medical Journal,* 1978, *71,* 340–342.

Surwit, R. S. Raynaud's disease. In L. Birk (Ed.), *Biofeedback: Behavioral medicine.* New York: Grune & Stratton, 1973.

Surwit, R. S., Allen, L. M., Kuhn, C. M., Gilgor, R. S., Duvic, M., Schandberg, S. M., & Williams, R. B. Neuroendocrine correlates of Raynaud's disease and phenomenon. *Psychophysiology,* 1981, *18,* 204. (Abstract)

Surwit, R. S., Bradner, M. B., Fenton, C. H., & Pilon, R. N. Individual differences in response to the behavioral treatment of Raynaud's disease. *Journal of Consulting and Clinical Psychology,* 1979, *47,* 363–367.

Surwit, R. S., & Fenton, C. H. Feedback and instructions in the control of digital skin temperature. *Psychophysiology,* 1980, *17,* 129–132.

Surwit, R. S., Pilon, R. N., & Fenton, C. H. Behavioral treatment of Raynaud's disease. *Journal of Behavioral Medicine,* 1978, *1,* 323–335.

Taub, E. Self regulation of human tissue temperature. In G. E. Schwartz & J. Beatty (Eds.), *Biofeedback: Theory and research.* New York: Academic Press, 1977.

Varadi, D. P., & Lawrence, A. M. Suppression of Raynaud's phenomenon by methyldopa. *Archives of Internal Medicine,* 1969, *124,* 13–18.

Wilkins, R. W., Doupe, J., & Newman, H. W. The rate of blood flow in normal fingers. *Clinical Science,* 1938, *3,* 403–411.

8

Migraine and Vascular Headache

Headache is an extremely complex phenomenon. Causes of head pain have been traced to such divergent sources as neoplasms, excessive muscle tension, ophthalmologic difficulties, neuralgias, cervical disc disease, sinusitis, and pain from distended and inflamed cerebral arteries (Diamond & Dalessio, 1978; Ryan & Ryan, 1978). It is this last form of headache, the vascular headache, that we will focus on in this chapter. Vascular headaches in and of themselves are attributable to a great variety of different syndromes. Although Graham and Wolff (1938) demonstrated that migraine headache is accompanied by vasodilatation of the cranial arteries, there are numerous reasons why such dilatation may occur. Vasodilatation can accompany toxic reactions, metabolic reactions, the presence of such vasodilator agents as histamine or nitrites, inflammation subsequent to concussion, inflammation subsequent to a convulsion, acute pressor reactions, or chronic essential hypertension (Lance, 1978). Of all the vascular-related headaches, it is the migraine headache that is the most common bane to the practicing physician. The term *migraine* refers to a specific type of headache that usually occurs unilaterally (hence, the term *migraine* meaning 'hemicranial'). Over the years, the definition of migraine has expanded to include bilateral headaches with features similar to the unilateral attacks. Typically, these headaches are preceded by neurological symptoms, such as scotomata, and are accompanied by nausea, vomiting, and photophobia. Headache onset may be sudden and severity variable. In general, the term *classic migraine* is reserved for those headaches that are strictly hemicranial and are accompanied by transient focal neurological phenomena followed by pounding pain, nausea, and vomiting. *Common* or *nonclassic migraine* is usually defined as general vascular headaches without focal neurological symptoms:

Headache pain may or may not be pounding, and nausea and vomiting do not have to be present.

PATHOPHYSIOLOGY OF MIGRAINE

It has long been known that extra- and intracranial vascular dilatation is an important component of the pain experienced in migraine (Graham & Wolff, 1938). In their classic experiment, Graham and Wolff administered ergotamine tartrate, a potent vasoconstrictor, to subjects during the painful phase of migraine while simultaneously recording extracranial vasomotor activity from the superficial temporal and occipital arteries. Upon administration of ergotamine, subjects showed a decrease in magnitude of pulse amplitudes ranging from 84% to 16%. This was accompanied by a corresponding decline in subjective headache intensity. Moreover, these investigators noted that headaches could be temporarily suppressed if manual pressure was exerted on the common carotid artery ipsolateral to the site of pain. Tunis and Wolff (1953) demonstrated that the magnitude of the temporal artery pulse of migraine sufferers was larger than that of non-migraine sufferers even when the patient population was asymptomatic. These investigators also noticed that migraine subjects showed considerable variability in pulse amplitude responses between 18 and 72 hr prior to the onset of the headache, with maximal amplitude variations occurring at the height of headache pain. This vascular instability has frequently been attributed to the autonomic nervous system. Appenzeller, Davison, and Marshall (1963) compared the reflex vasomotor responses in the hands of migraine subjects with similar responses in the hands of headache-free subjects. They noted that, whereas normal subjects showed forearm vasodilatation in response to heating of the lower extremities, this response was absent in 8 out of 10 migraine subjects. However, other experimenters have failed to replicate this finding (e.g., French, Lassers, & DeSai, 1967).

While these data imply a relationship between autonomic nervous system activity and migraine, the situation is far more complicated than that of Raynaud's disease and peripheral vasospastic disorders. First, unlike the arterioles of the digits, which have no active neurogenic vasodilatory mechanisms, the arterioles in the brain will vasodilate in response to beta adrenergic stimulation. Other neurotransmitters found in the central nervous system (CNS) may play an important role in the production of migraine. Anthony, Hinterberger, and Lance (1967) and Curran, Hinterberger, and Lance (1965) have noted blood levels of serotonin, a potent vasoconstrictor, rise slightly before the onset of a migraine and then fall sharply with the arrival of pain. Plasma serotonin then tends to increase after vomiting and diarrhea, and this has often been reported to accompany relief of headache pain. Interestingly, it has often been noted that injection of reserpine, which lowers plasma serotonin levels, often produces a dull headache in nonmigraine sufferers and a typical migraine in migraineurs. Intravenous injection of serotonin in spontaneous or reserpine-induced migraines increases plasma serotonin and alleviates headache (Anthony *et al.*, 1967). Migraine sufferers have also been shown to be unduly sensitive to insulin and blood glucose levels. In addition to serotonin, histamine, bradykinen, monoaminoxydase, as well as prostaglandins have been implicated in migraine activity (Lance, 1978).

Although the pathophysiology of migraine is more complex than that of peripheral vascular disease, it is clear that the autonomic nervous system plays some role in the phenomenon of migraine. Hsu, Crisp, Koval, Kalway, Chem, Carruthers, and Zilka (1976) studied patients whose headaches awaken them from sleep. They noted that plasma norepinephrine was significantly elevated in the 3 hr preceding the headache, which commonly occurred during the rapid eye movement (REM) phase of sleep. This same change in plasma norepinephrine was not found in normals during REM sleep. Fog-Moller, Genefke, and Bryndum (1976) noted that, once a headache is established, plasma levels of norepinephrine decline and reach a minimum value 1.5 hr prior to peak headache pain, rising again as headache intensity eases. Because norepinephrine constricts the arterioles and capillaries, it is of interest that the sensitivity of these vessels to the topical application of norepinephrine increases during the prodromal phase and decreases during the headache itself (Ostfeld & Wolff, 1955). As with infusion of serotonin, Wolff (1972) noted that infusions of norepinephrine also alleviate the headache. If norepinephrine was infused in headache-free periods for up to 3 hr and then abruptly discontinued, no headache ensued. Thus, it appears unlikely that migraine is simply a reactive hyperemia following tissue ischemia due to excessive sympathetic nervous system activity.

PSYCHOLOGICAL CHARACTERISTICS

The traditional psychosomatic literature is replete with characterizations of the migraine personality. The stereotype of the migraine sufferer is that of a "tense, driving, obsessional perfectionist, with an inflexible personality, who maintains a store of bottled up resentments which neither can be expressed nor resolved" [Henryk-Gutt & Rees, p. 142, 1973]." The headache is thus thought to result from suppressed hostility that the migraine sufferer cannot express behaviorally. Bakal (1975) notes, however, that despite prevalence of this view there are very few objective studies utilizing control groups and psychometric tests to confirm this hypothesis. The only comprehensive attempt at such an assessment was performed by Henryk-Gutt and Rees (1973). Using the Eysenck Personality Inventory, the Minnesota Multiphasic Personality Inventory, the Buss-Durkee Hostility–Guilt Inventory, and careful diagnostic classifications (classic migraines, common migraines, and nonmigraine headache sufferers, a control group of headache-free subjects, migraine subjects attending a clinic, and asthma subjects), these investigators found that all migraine subjects had higher neuroticism and obsessional scores (Eysenck Personality Inventory) than controls did. Only the classic migraine male subjects and the female migraine subjects attending the clinics were significantly higher than control subjects on hostility as measured by the Buss-Durkee scale. Also, Bakal points out that the behavioral manifestation of these personality traits tends to be quite idiosyncratic. He argues that this combined with the inconsistency of reported personality traits associated with migraine detracts from the clinical impression that there is a definite migrainous personality. While migraine sufferers may in general appear to be somewhat more neurotic, this may in part be explained by their chronic physical condition, which is responsive to stress.

Lance (1978) has attempted to summarize the interaction of all contributing factors in the development and maintenance of vascular headaches (see Figure 8.1). In this schema, the cranial vascular system is regarded as the end organ of the pain process. During a headache, blood is shunted away from the periphery, causing pallor in the case of the extracranial vascular tree and focal neurological symptoms resulting from cortical ischemia in the case of intracranial vessels. He postulates an enhanced, possibly an inherited, tendency of vascular contractility in migrainous patients. This could be aggravated by autonomic, humoral, or immune factors. Serotonin, which can be released from the platelets in migraine, is seen to cause vasoconstriction. In combination with histamine and kinens, it is then absorbed into the vessel wall, increasing the sensitivity of the arteries to pain. The increased blood flow that follows may be a reactive hyperemia or a response to specific vasodilator agents. Additional postulated metabolic changes in migraine include sodium and fluid retention, abnormal glucose metabolism, and elevation of free fatty acids. Pain is seen as resulting from distension of the vasculature as well as from increased sensitivity of the vascular wall. While migraines may be stimulated by changes in internal brain chemistry, Lance believes that they are more commonly caused by external trigger factors, physical or emotional, that operate through the autonomic nervous system, humoral agents, or immune mechanisms. "The end result is a neurovascular reaction which reduces the blood supply to the vulnerable parts of the brain with results detrimental to the patient. The headache, itself, like any form of pain which signals a threat to bodily function, may be a byproduct

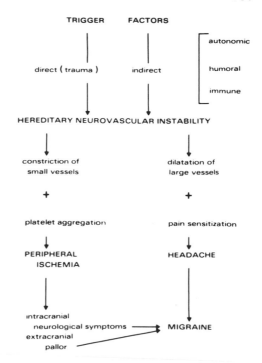

TRIGGER   FACTORS

direct (trauma)   indirect

autonomic

humoral

immune

HEREDITARY NEUROVASCULAR INSTABILITY

constriction of
small vessels

dilatation of
large vessels

+

+

platelet aggregation

pain sensitization

PERIPHERAL
ISCHEMIA

HEADACHE

intracranial
neurological symptoms
extracranial
pallor

MIGRAINE

FIGURE 8.1. Factors in the pathogenesis of migraine. [From J. W. Lance. *Mechanism and Management of Migraine* (3rd ed.). (London: Butterworth, 1978, p. 173).]

of such reactions, even though it represents the major problem to the patient [Lance, 1978, p. 177]."

MEDICAL TREATMENT OF MIGRAINE

The medical treatment of migraine encompasses the use of most techniques used in medical practice. Pharmacotherapy, manipulation, and surgery have all been tried with varying results. Surgical management has usually involved operation on sympathetic or parasympathetic nerves and ligation of the branches of the external carotid or meningal arteries. Neither procedure has been very effective (Lance, 1978). Pharmacotherapy has involved the use of numerous substances, from narcotics and analgesics to antidepressants. Narcotics and analgesics, because they relieve the pain of the headache, have become the most often used, and abused, medications in the treatment of migraine (Diamond, 1979). Unfortunately, patients tend to habituate to the effects of these medications, requiring higher doses of each drug and frequent changes from one analgesic to another (Diamond, 1979). More specific therapy

for migraine is available from ergotamine tartrate. Ergotamine was used in
Europe as early as 1883 (Diamond, 1979), although its specific vasoconstrictive effects were not known until Graham and Wolff published their now
classic study. It remains one of the most potent treatments available for the
acute episode (Lance, 1978). The list of pharmacologic interventions is ency-
clopedic. Vasodilators (such as clonidine and reserpine), beta-adrenergic blocking agents (such as propranolol), monamine oxidase inhibitors, tricyclic antidepressants, anticonvulsants, prostoglandin antagonists, antihistamines, and
sex hormones have all been used with varying success in the treatment of
chronic migraine (Lance, 1978). None of these regimens has proven itself
universally effective, and many patients fail to respond to any of these treatments (Graham, 1979).

BEHAVIORAL TREATMENT OF MIGRAINE

Recent interest in the application of behavioral techniques to the treatment
of migraine headache can be traced to the early work of Sargent, Green, and
Walters (1972). These investigators reported on a subject who was learning to
relax by reducing electromyographic (EMG) potential in the forearm and increasing skin temperature in the digits of the hand. The investigators reported
that spontaneous recovery from a migraine was correlated with a 10°F increase
in digital skin temperature over a 2-min period during relaxation. They then
reasoned that, if a "spontaneous" increase in skin temperature was associated
with headache relief, then inducing digital vasodilatation voluntarily may provide a behavioral treatment of migraine. Although this rationale has dubious
logical face validity, it led to the development of a whole literature on the use
of skin temperature feedback, usually accompanied by some form of relaxation
instruction, as a treatment for migraine.

Biofeedback

The first of these reports (Sargent et al., 1972) involved 42 subjects. These
subjects were trained to increase the temperature of the right index finger
relative to the midforehead. All subjects were given autogenic instructions and
asked to practice daily with a portable temperature feedback device. Subjects
were first seen at weekly intervals and then on a less frequent basis. The length
of treatment varied from 3 weeks to 3 months, and all subjects returned inter-
mittently to the clinic for at least 1 year. As in many of the later reports on the
use of digital temperature training as a treatment for migraine, no data were
provided as to the ability of subjects to raise temperature or on the relationship

between this ability and clinical improvement. Thirty-four of the original 42 subjects (81%) were rated to be improved. Of these subjects, 9 reported a slight improvement, 9 a moderate improvement, 10 a good improvement, and 6 a very good improvement (able to abort headaches and eliminate the need for medication). Subsequent publications by this group (e.g., Sargent, Walters, & Green, 1973; Solback & Sargent, 1977) have added subjects to this original patient pool to increase the number to 74.

Wickramasekera (1973) reported on two subjects whom he treated with EMG feedback and then digital skin temperature feedback without autogenic phrases. Although this report contains a very small number of subjects, both of them were seen to increase digital temperature greater than 5°F during training. The subjects received 16 and 18 sessions of EMG training followed by 10 and 11 weeks of temperature training. At a 3-month follow-up, both subjects were headache free and had significantly reduced medication intake. Turin and Johnson (1976) reported on one subject who received first instructions to lower digital temperature using digital skin temperature feedback and later instructions to raise temperature using the same feedback procedure. The subject was given 12 sessions of temperature feedback to decrease skin temperature and 12 sessions of temperature feedback to increase skin temperature. During the first phase of training, the subject reported a slight increase in headache frequency as compared to baseline. During the second phase of training, the subject was able to raise skin temperature up to 4°F during sessions and reported a slight decrease in the number and frequency of headaches over baseline. Adler and Adler (1976) reported on training 22 patients suffering from migraine headache with a combination of EMG feedback followed by digital skin temperature feedback. The number of sessions ranged from 5 to 60. These authors reported that 81% of their patients showed at least a 75% reduction in the frequency of headaches in a 3.5-year follow-up period. In a similar design Medina, Diamond, and Franklin (1976) treated 13 migraine patients with both EMG and temperature feedback. All subjects were leased a home temperature feedback trainer for a 1-month period and given autogenic phrases to use at home. Subjects were then seen on a follow-up basis once every 2 months for a period of 6–33 months. Nine of the 14 subjects showed at least a 30% reduction in headache frequency. All subjects were found to have maintained their gains at follow-up. All subjects were able to show voluntary hand temperature increases of at least 2°F at the last feedback session.

Reading and Mohr (1976) reported on the use of skin temperature feedback in six migrainous subjects who had been resistant to drug treatment. This study is of interest because it was more systematic than those previously reported. During the first phase of each session, subjects were given a brief stabilization period before training began. During the second phase, subjects were given three 7-min periods during which time they were told to try to increase their digital skin temperature using feedback. During the third phase, subjects sat quietly without feedback. All subjects were encouraged to practice hand warming at home without the aid of a feedback device. All subjects reported to be able to raise their temperature voluntarily at least 1.4°C even without feedback. Also, all subjects reported a mean decrease in headache frequency from 4.1 per week pretreatment to 1.9 per week posttreatment. The duration of these headaches was reduced by approximately 60%. Prior to treatment, subjects reported a total of 25.3 hr of headaches per week as compared to a total of 10.4 hr following treatment. At 2-month follow-up, subjects were reporting an average of 1 headache per week lasting approximately 5 hr. Mitch, McGrady, and Iannone (1976) conducted a systematic multiple baseline investigation on 20 subjects suffering from migraine headaches. In their study, all subjects were exposed to three phases of treatment. In phase 1, lasting 4 weeks, subjects were given digital skin temperature feedback and autogenic instructions and asked to practice finger warming at home on a regular basis. Subjects met with the therapist every 2 weeks. In phase 2, also lasting 4 weeks, the subjects were asked to continue practicing on a regular basis but also to use their new strategy whenever a headache occurred. In phase 3, regular practice was discontinued and subjects were asked to continue using finger warming if headaches occurred. Unfortunately, the authors do not report the extent to which subjects were able to increase digital temperature. As in many other studies, their ratings of improvement were global. Sixty-five percent of all subjects were rated improved on at least two measures of intensity, frequency, duration, or medication use. Half of the subjects reported in for follow-ups 6 months later. All of them had maintained their initial gains.

These studies fail to make a conclusive argument for the use of skin temperature feedback in the treatment of migraine headaches. Although Sargent, Walters, and Green (1973) hypothesized that their technique worked by reducing general sympathetic outflow, this, of course, provides little rationale for their differential temperature feedback method. However, these authors have abandoned differential feedback in their more recent work in favor of feedback from the digit alone. It is unfortunate that none of the previously cited studies reports on the effect of skin temperature training on other autonomic responses (e.g., galvanic skin response (GSR), heart rate, blood pressure, etc.) Only the Turin and Johnson (1976) and Johnson and Turin (1975) studies, by training subjects to increase and decrease hand temperature in distinct phases of treatment, relate temperature increases or the subject's attempt to produce these increases with an improvement in headache frequency.

The first attempt at a controlled group outcome study was that of Andreychuk and Skriver (1975). Twenty-eight subjects were assigned to one of three treatment conditions: training in self-hypnosis, emphasizing relaxation and visual imagery, and instructions on dealing with pain; hand temperature training (audiofeedback) and autogenic training; and training in the production of the electroencephalogram (EEG) alpha with audiofeedback. All subjects were given one 45-min training session per week for 10 weeks. The most interesting result of this study is that the highly hypnotizable subjects showed the greatest improvement. Differences between treatment groups were not significant. Kondo and Canter (1977) trained 20 subjects in a two-group experiment. The first group was given frontalis EMG feedback without specific relaxation instructions. The second group was given false frontalis EMG feedback. After 10 20-min sessions, the authors noted greater decreases in EMG in the true feedback group than in the false feedback group. In addition, the group receiving true feedback decreased their mean number of headaches for a 5-day block from 5.2 to 1. Interestingly, the group receiving false feedback also showed a decrease in headache frequency from 4.5 to 3.5. This difference was reported to be statistically significant. At 12-month follow-up, half of the subjects in each group were recontacted; 80% of the subjects in the true feedback group reported maintaining gains, whereas no subjects in the false feedback group could be rated as significantly improved. Philips (1977) trained 15 subjects in a similar design. Eight subjects received true frontalis or temporalis feedback. The other group received false feedback from the same muscle group. Subjects in the false feedback group were told that the clicking sound of the EMG feedback would help them relax. All subjects received two sessions a week for 6 weeks. As in the study by Kondo and Canter, subjects receiving true EMG feedback showed decreases in that response, whereas no decreases were shown in the group receiving false feedback. Subjects receiving true EMG feedback reported a 30% drop in headache frequency, whereas subjects receiving false feedback reported a 16% drop. However, unlike the study by Kondo and Canter, differences between the two groups were not statistically significant. At follow-up 6–8 weeks later, subjects who had received true feedback showed further headache reductions, whereas the group receiving false feedback did not change. Significant group differences were found on measures of headache intensity, with the true feedback group decreasing headache intensity up to 50% from baseline and no change in the group receiving false feedback.

Blanchard, Theobald, Williamson, Silver, and Brown (1978) applied a controlled group outcome design to test differential efficacy of temperature biofeedback as compared to progressive relaxation or a waiting-list control. Ten subjects were given temperature feedback with autogenic training, and 10 subjects were given progressive muscle relaxation training. Both groups were encouraged to practice at home. Ten subjects constituted a waiting-list control. Subjects in both the temperature feedback and relaxation conditions showed significantly greater decreases in frequency and intensity than did the waiting-list control subjects. Interestingly, subjects receiving progressive relaxation did slightly better than subjects receiving temperature feedback and autogenic training. At a 1-month follow-up, the gains were maintained in 9 out of 13 in the group receiving temperature feedback and in all the subjects receiving relaxation training. These differences were not statistically significant.

Mullinix, Morton, Hack, and Fishman (1978) divided 12 subjects into two treatment conditions. Half of the subjects received true temperature feedback from the middle digit of the dominant hand, while half of the subjects received false temperature feedback. All subjects were given six 30-min training sessions and were instructed to practice at home. While skin temperature data were inadequately reported, the authors did indicate that true temperature feedback subjects obtained significantly greater mean temperature increases than did false feedback subjects. There was little correlation between temperature changes and clinical results. There were no significant differences between the two treatment groups as to outcome. Approximately half of the subjects in both groups showed reductions in headache severity.

Price and Tursky (1976) measured peripheral vascular activity in the digit and in the temporal artery using photoplethysmography in 40 female migraine patients and 49 matched controls. In the migraine patients, the photoplethysmograph was positioned ipsilateral to the pain site or on the left side if headaches were bilateral. Subjects in both groups were assigned to one of four training conditions: continuous visual blood volume feedback; false yoked feedback; relaxation training without feedback; or a neutral tape recording (instructions on how to grow a plant). Only one training session was used. In this session, the first two groups were instructed to try to increase hand temperature and the remaining two were instructed to listen to the relaxation or the botany instructions, which they were told would help them increase hand temperature. While normal subjects were able to increase blood volume in the hand with feedback, the migraine patients tended to show no change in hand temperature with or without feedback. Koppman, McDonald, and Kunzel (1974) demonstrated that migraine patients could produce voluntary vasodilatation or constriction of the superficial temporal artery using a similar reflectance technique. No correlation was found between these changes and simultaneously recorded finger blood flow or masseter muscle activity.

Friar and Beatty (1976) assigned 19 female patients suffering from migraine to one of two conditions. The first group was given visual and auditory feedback to reduce pulse amplitude over the extracranial artery of the most affected side. The second group was trained to reduce pulse amplitude in the index finger of the most affected side. Subjects provided with feedback of finger pulse amplitude succeeded in reducing the amplitude by 67% of baseline without producing a corresponding change in temporal artery pulse amplitude. However, the group given cephalic pulse amplitude training showed an 80% change from baseline and a corresponding decrease in the amplitude of the digital pulse. Subjects given temporal artery pulse feedback showed a significant decrease in the total number of headache episodes. Subjects given digital pulse amplitude feedback showed a smaller and nonsignificant decrease.

Bild and Adams (1980) compared the efficacy of cephalic blood volume feedback with EMG frontalis feedback and a waiting-list control. Seven subjects were given 10 sessions of training to reduce the amplitude of temporal artery pulse, while six subjects were given 10 sessions of EMG frontalis feedback. The instructions for both groups of subjects were identical except for the directions concerning their specific response training. The group trained in temporal artery vasoconstriction was told to constrict "the temporal arteries by turning off the tone," while the EMG group was told to "turn off the tone by relaxation of the frontalis muscles." An additional six subjects constituted a waiting-for-treatment control, during which time they recorded headache activity and medication intake. Subjects being given temporal artery pulse amplitude feedback were able to decrease the amplitude of this response voluntarily. Subjects given EMG feedback were able to show some control over this variable. While all subjects tended to decrease headache frequency over the 6 weeks of initial observation, the decrease was significantly greater for those subjects receiving temporal artery pulse amplitude feedback than for those receiving EMG feedback. However, at an 18-week follow-up there were no statistically significant differences between groups. Although the authors claim that subjects receiving temporal artery pulse amplitude decreased the use of sedatives and vasoconstrictive medications more than those receiving EMG feedback or no treatment at all, they do not report whether or not these results were statistically significant.

Sovak, Kunzel, Sternbach, and Dalessio (1978) trained 5 normal volunteers and 12 migraine subjects to raise their hand temperature with the use of autogenic training and skin temperature feedback. All subjects received eight 45-min sessions over a 4-week period. Ability to raise skin temperature voluntarily was defined as the ability to raise temperature 2°C within 15 min in the laboratory. All of the normal subjects and 10 of the 12 migraineurs learned to raise their hand temperature to this criterion. Of the 10 migraine patients, 8 reported a 50% reduction in headache frequency and intensity and were therefore rated as improved. In addition, it was observed that voluntarily increasing skin temperature in both normals and migraine patients was accompanied by a decrease in blood flow to the frontal and temporal regions. Average supraorbital pulse amplitude was significantly decreased in both normals and migraineurs, whereas average temporal artery pulse amplitude was significantly reduced in normals and insignificantly reduced in migraineurs. Unimproved migraineurs showed no change in supraorbital artery or temporal artery pulse amplitude. To test the notion that changes in extracranial pulse amplitude might be a result of hemodynamic redistribution following peripheral vasodilatation, the hands of both normal and migraine subjects were exposed to a current of 85°C air. In normal subjects this was accompanied by an increase in the pulse volume of both the supraorbital and temporal artery vascular beds. However, in improved migraineurs there was a decrease in temporal artery pulse amplitude and an insignificant decrease in supraorbital artery pulse amplitude. In another study, Largen, Mathew, Dobbins, Meyer, and Claghorn (1978) trained 12 normal female subjects to increase or decrease the skin temperature of their hands. Following extensive training, regional cerebral blood flow was measured during a relaxation period and also when subjects were self-regulating skin temperature. While the skin temperatures of the hand-warming and the hand-cooling groups changed significantly in opposite directions, there were no related changes in the regional cerebral blood flow.

Relaxation and Other Techniques

Although the initial interest in behavioral treatment of headaches stemmed from the application of biofeedback techniques to this disorder, it is becoming increasingly clear that techniques other than biofeedback can be used in the treatment of headaches. For instance, Hay and Madders (1971) reported on a series of 98 patients suffering from migraines who were treated with progressive muscle relaxation. Although the report is not well documented, they claim that nearly two-thirds of their patient population improved with training. Paulley and Haskell (1975) report an even larger success rate in a series of over 800 patients. Like Hay and Madders, Paulley and Haskell provide no clear documentation to evaluate their results. However, on an anecdotal level, they claim that three-fourths of their patient population demonstrated long-term success with training. These results seem credible in light of the studies of Blanchard *et al.* in which relaxation training was shown to be superior to skin temperature feedback.

Mitchell has published a series of studies that demonstrate the use of a wide range of behavioral techniques in the treatment of headaches. Mitchell and Mitchell (1971) reported that the use of systematic desensitization when added to relaxation training could significantly augment the treatment effects of the latter. Those patients treated with systematic desensitization demonstrated a 76% reduction in migraine frequency and a 50% reduction in duration of each headache, compared with a 24% reduction in frequency and no reduction in duration of headache for those patients treated with relaxation only. In a study of 12 migraine patients, Mitchell and White (1977) used a multiple baseline design to which a variety of behavioral techniques were added over time. In the first stage of this study, all 12 patients engaged only in the recording of headache frequency, duration, medication consumption, etc. for a 12-week period. Three groups of subjects (N = 9) were then trained and required to self-record and monitor the circumstances preceding the onset of migraine headaches. Following the end of the 12-week period, group 2 continued to monitor headaches and situational stimuli for headaches, while groups 3 and 4 proceeded to another skill. The results are shown in Figure 8.2. The skill acquisition training packages involved cue controlled progressive muscle relaxation, mental and differential relaxation, and self-desensitization. In stage 2, more advanced and complicated versions of similar techniques were presented. Mitchell and White (1977) conclude that effective behavioral treatment of headaches must take into account all factors in the production of migraine and that training must teach patients to cope actively with stress in an adaptive

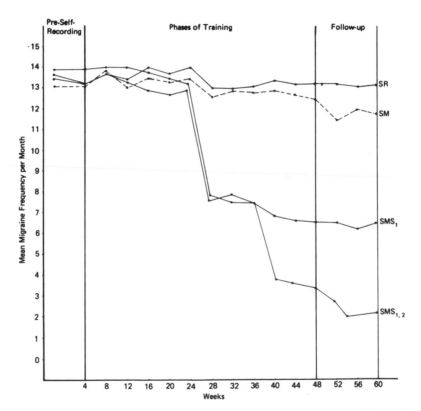

FIGURE 8.2. Changes in migraine frequency with increments to training in behavioral self-management. SR = self-recording only; SM = self-monitoring only; SMS_1 = self-recording, self-monitoring, and skill acquisition stage 1; $SMS_{1,2}$ = self-recording, self-monitoring, and skill acquisition stages 1 and 2. [From K. R. Mitchell & R. G. White. Behavioral self-management: An application to the problem of migraine headaches. *Behavior Therapy*, 1977, 8, 219.]

way. It is unfortunate that this study used such a small number of subjects, because its rationale has a lot of face validity.

CONCLUSION

In summary, it seems clear that, as Adams, Feurestein, and Fowler (1980) pointed out, while psychoanalysis and psychodynamic therapy have been of very limited value in the treatment of migraine, behavioral approaches appear more promising. Because biofeedback techniques make up the bulk of this behavioral literature, there is more persuasive evidence for their efficacy than for the efficacy of other procedures. However, comparative studies offer few data to support the advantage of one technique over another. Although Yates (1980) justifiably calls the technical standard of research in the area "deplorably poor in quality [p. 247]," the sheer volume of the studies and case reports that claim clinical efficacy argue persuasively that behavioral techniques have something to offer in the treatment of vascular headaches.

What can be concluded from these studies? First of all, it appears that there is no simple hemodynamic redistribution that takes place when subjects are taught to increase skin temperature with biofeedback, relaxation, or other techniques. Largen *et al.* (1978) could find no relationship between direction of change of hand temperature and regional cerebral blood flow. Although Sovak *et al.* (1978) did observe that voluntarily increasing hand temperature was accompanied by a decrease in extracranial blood flow to the frontal and temporal regions, they conclude that the vasomotor pathophysiology in vascular headaches is so variable that no single hemodynamic redistribution of cardiac output can be seen to be specifically active in explaining the effects of behavioral training. Because they found that vasoconstriction in the extracranial superficial arteries is more easily elicited in migraineurs than in normals, they hypothesize that skin temperature feedback may work by reducing a heightened sympathetic tone, which they claim is characteristic of the migraine population. This notion is supported by Appenzeller (1969), who has noted that migraineurs are known to have intermittent prolonged periods of sympathetic outflow. In addition, Price and Tursky (1976) have also observed the exaggerated tendency of migraine patients to display cerebral vasoconstriction. Thus, it appears plausible to assume that, for one reason or another, migraine subjects do show a high degree of cerebral vascular lability that is mediated in part by the activity of the sympathetic nervous system. It would, therefore, follow that any behavioral technique that can cause a reduction in sympathetic nervous system activity might be beneficial to the migraine patient. It would, also, appear that the elevated skin temperature found to accompany relaxation or skin temperature feedback training in the treatment of a migraine syndrome represents a decrease in general sympathetic outflow, which produces a reduction in migraine symptoms by minimizing cerebral vascular instability. Other behavioral procedures that have a similar effect on the autonomic nervous system should logically also be effective in the management of migraine. The current literature on the behavioral treatment of migraine suggests that this is the case.

REFERENCES

Adams, H., Feuerstein, M., & Fowler, J. Migraine headache: Review of parameters, etiology and intervention. *Psychological Bulletin*, 1980, 87, 217–237.

Adler, C., & Adler, S. Biofeedback-psychotherapy for the treatment of headaches: A five year clinical follow-up. *Headache*, 1976, 16, 189–191.

Andreychuk, T., & Skriver, C. Hypnosis and biofeedback in the treatment of migraine headache. *International Journal of Clinical and Experimental Hypnosis*, 1975, 23, 172–183.

Anthony, M., Hinterberger, H., & Lance, J. W. Plasma serotonin in migraine and stress. *Archives of Neurology*, 16: 544–552, 1967.

Appenzeller, D. Vasomotor function in migraine. *Headache*, 1969, 9, 147–155.

Appenzeller, D., Davison, K., & Marshall, J. Reflex vasomotor abnormalities in the hands of migrainous subjects. *Journal of Neurosurgery and Psychiatry*, 1963, 26, 447.

Bakal, D. A. Headache: A biopsychological perspective. *Psychological Bulletin*, 1975, 82, 369–382.

Bild, R., & Adams, H. E. Modification of migraine headache by cephalic blood volume pulse and EMG biofeedback. *Journal of Consulting and Clinical Psychology*, 1980, 48, 51–57.

Blanchard, E. B., Theobald, D., Williamson, D., Silver, B., & Brown, B. Temperature feedback in the treatment of migraine headaches. *Archives of General Psychology*, 1978, 35, 581–588.

Curran, D. A., Hinterberger, H., & Lance, J. W. Total plasma serotonin, 5-hydroxyindoleacetic acid and p-hydroxy-m-methoxymandelic acid excretion in normal and migrainous subjects. *Brain*, 1965, 88, 997–1010.

Diamond, S. Panel discussion: The use of analgesics in headache. *Headache*, 1979, 19, 185–190.

Diamond, S., & Dalessio, D. J. *The practicing physician's approach to headache* (2nd ed.), Baltimore: Williams & Wilkins, 1978.

Fog-Moller, F., Genefke, I. K., & Bryndum, B. Changes in concentration of catecholamines in blood during spontaneous migraine attacks and reserpine induced attacks. *Abstracts International Symposium*, September 16–17, p. 10, London: Migraine Trust, 1976.

French, E. B., Lassers, B. W., & DeSai, M. G. Reflex vasomotor responses in the hands of migrainous subjects. *Journal of Neurology, Neurosurgery and Psychiatry*, 1967, 30, 276–278.

Friar, L. R., & Beatty, J. Migraine: Management by trained control of vasoconstriction. *Journal of Consulting and Clinical Psychology*, 1976, 44, 46–53.

Graham, J. R. Migraine headache: Diagnosis and Management. *Headache*, 1979, 19, 133–141.

Graham, J. R., & Wolff, H. G. Mechanism of migraine headache and action of ergotamine tartrate. *Archives of Neurological Psychiatry*, 1938, 39, 737–763.

Hay, K. M., & Madders, J. Migraine treated by relaxation therapy. *Journal of the Royal College of General Practitioners*, 1971, 21, 664–669.

Henryk-Gutt, R., & Rees, W. L. Psychological aspects of migraine. *Journal of Psychosomatic Research*, 1973, 17, 141–153.

Hsu, L. G. U., Crisp, A. H., Koval J., Kalway, R. S., Chem, C. M., Carruthers, M., & Zilka, K. Electroencephalogram and plasma levels of catecholamines, tryptophan, glucose, insulin, insulin free fatty acids and prostaglandins during sleep preceding early-morning migraine. *International Symposium*, September 16–17, p. 11, London: Migraine Trust, 1976.

Johnson, W. G., & Turin, A. Biofeedback treatment of migraine headache: A systematic case study. *Behavior Therapy*, 1975, *6*, 394–397.

Kondo, C., & Canter, A. True and False electromyographic feedback: Effect on tension headache. *Journal of Abnormal Psychology*, 1977, *86*, 93–95.

Koppman, J. W., McDonald, R. D., & Kunzel, M. G. Voluntary regulation of temporal artery diameter in migraine patients. *Headache*, 1974, *14*, 133–138.

Lance, J. W. *Mechanism and management of headache* (3rd ed.). Boston: Butterworths, 1978.

Largen, J. W., Mathew, R. J., Dobbins, K., Meyer, J. S., & Claghorn, J. L. Skin temperature self-regulation and non-invasive regional cerebral blood flow. *Headache*, 1978, *18*, 203–210.

Medina, J. L., Diamond, S., & Franklin, M. A. Biofeedback therapy for migraine. *Headache*, 1976, *16*, 115–118.

Mitch, P. S., McGrady, A., & Iannone, A. Autogenic feedback in migraine: A treatment report. *Headache*, 1976, *15*, 267–270.

Mitchell, K. R., & Mitchell, D. M. Migraine: An exploratory treatment application of programmed behavior therapy techniques. *Journal of Psychosomatic Research*, 1971, *15*, 137–157.

Mitchell, K. R., & White, R. G. Behavioral self-management: An application to the problem of migraine headaches. *Behavior Therapy*, 1977, *8*, 213–221.

Mullinix, J., Morton, B., Hack, S., & Fishman, M. Skin temperature biofeedback and migraine. *Headache*, 1978, *17*, 242–244.

Ostfeld, A. M., & Wolff, H. G. Studies on headache: Arteriolar (norepinephrine) and vascular headache of the migraine type. *Archives of Neurological Psychiatry*, 1955, *74*, 131–136.

Paulley, J. W., & Haskell, D. A. L. The treatment of migraine without drugs. *Journal of Psychosomatic Research*, 1975, *19*, 367–374.

Philips, C. The modification of tension headache pain using EMG biofeedback. *Behavior Research and Therapy*, 1977, *15*, 119–129.

Price, K. P., & Tursky, B. Vascular reactivity of migraineurs and non-migraineurs: A comparison of responses to self control procedures. *Headache*, 1976, *16*, 210–217.

Reading, C., & Mohr, P. D. Biofeedback control of migraine: A pilot study. *British Journal of Social and Clinical Psychology*, 1976, *15*, 429–433.

Ryan, R. E., Sr., & Ryan, R. E., Jr. *Headache and head pain: Diagnosis and treatment*. St. Louis: Mosby, 1978.

Sargent, J. D., Green, E. E., & Walters, E. D. The use of autogenic feedback training in a pilot study of migraine and tension headaches. *Headache*, 1972, *12*, 120–125.

Sargent, J. D., Green, E. E., & Walters, E. D. Preliminary report on the use of autogenic feedback training in the treatment of migraine and tension headaches. *Psychosomatic Medicine*, 1973, *35*, 129–135. (*a*)

Sargent, J. D., Walters, E. D., & Green, E. E. Psychosomatic self-regulation of migraine headaches. In L. Birk (Ed.), *Biofeedback: Behavioral medicine*. New York: Grune & Stratton, 1973. (*b*)

Solback, A. P., & Sargent, J. D. Follow-up evaluation of the Menninger pilot migraine study using thermal training. *Headache*, 1977, *17*, 198–202.

Sovak, M., Kunzel, M., Sternbach, R. A., & Dalessio, D. J. Is volitional manipulation of hemodynamics a valid rationale for biofeedback therapy of migraine? *Headache*, 1978, *18*, 197–202.

Tunis, M. M., & Wolff, H. G. Analysis of cranial artery pulse waves in migraine type. *American Journal of Medical Science*, 1953, *224*, 565–568.

Turin, A., & Johnson, W. G. Biofeedback therapy for migraine headache. *Archives of General Psychiatry,* 1976, 33, 517–519.

Wickramasekera, I. Temperature feedback for the control of migraine. *Journal of Behavior Therapy and Experimental Psychiatry,* 1973, *4,* 343–345.

Wolff, H. G. *Headache and other head pain* (3rd ed. Revised by D. J. Dalessio). New York: Oxford University Press, 1972.

Yates, A. J. *Biofeedback and the modification of behavior.* New York: Plenum, 1980.

9

Clinical Issues in the Application of Behavioral Techniques in the Treatment of Disease

In the preceding chapters, we have discussed the rationale and the application of behavioral techniques in the treatment of a variety of cardiovascular disorders. Although behavioral techniques can be shown experimentally to produce therapeutic changes in many different disease states, a wide variety of clinical issues must be considered in order for therapy to be practical and effective. Up until now we have been discussing the application of behavioral techniques in much the same way as we would have discussed the use of a new drug or surgical procedure. However, it must be always kept in mind that when dealing with behavioral interventions treatment really consists of training. This is more than a subtle distinction, for it implies an active role on the patient's part, which is often in sharp contrast to the passive role that most conventional forms of medical treatment place the subject in. This distinction has numerous implications for the professional and the patient seeking help. In this chapter, we hope to call the reader's attention to the salient aspects of this issue.

COST-EFFECTIVENESS

One immediate difference between behavioral interventions and most conventional forms of medical treatment is the amount of time a therapist (professional or paraprofessional) must spend with a patient in order to achieve a therapeutic outcome. Whereas many medical problems can be handled with a 15-min consultation and surgical procedures accomplished in several hours, the demand that behavioral training makes upon both the patients' and the therapists' time may be considerable. How much time and effort, on the part of both patient and practitioner, is needed to obtain a clinically beneficial result? Even if the behavioral techniques can be shown to be highly efficacious, what patient would opt for a costly, time-consuming course of treatment if equal therapeutic benefit could be obtained from medications costing 10–20 cents a day? There is no simple answer to this question, but there are several rules of thumb that one can use to assess the practicality of behavioral intervention for each particular disorder. First of all, is a safe and effective medical or surgical alternative possible? If one is, then a good reason for wanting to use a behavioral approach must exist. Hypertension, while an attractive target for behavioral intervention on theoretical grounds, may be a poor candidate for treatment from a practical standpoint. Many hypertensive patients can be effectively managed with one or possibly two medications that are often without significant side effects and are relatively inexpensive. Except for the patients who cannot tolerate medication, there would seem to be little reason to substitute behavioral training for conventional medical therapy. However, in the case of Raynaud's disease and migraine headache, for example, there is no uniformly effective medical or surgical remedy available. Thus, behavioral techniques are much more attractive comparatively.

The cost-effectiveness of a behavioral intervention also depends upon the number and length of training sessions the patient must attend, the amount of professional time that must go into those training sessions, and the amount of expensive equipment required in the training. While it is generally conceded that the interpersonal skill of a therapist is as important in behavioral approaches as it is in psychodynamic approaches (Lanyon & Lanyon, 1978; Lynn & Freedman, 1979), it is not necessary to employ doctoral-level personnel in the administration of behavior therapy techniques (Ryback & Surwit, 1971). Paraprofessionals trained in the administration of relaxation, biofeedback, and contingency management procedures can, under the supervision of professional personnel, provide an efficient means of care delivery.

In addition to using paraprofessional personnel in health care delivery, there are many ways in which behavioral methods can be made economically feasible alternatives of two existing medical treatments. Surwit and Keefe (1978) have noted that the use of electromyographic (EMG) biofeedback, while not necessarily superior to progressive muscle relaxation, does provide an effective way of automating the delivery of relaxation training to large numbers of patients. Biofeedback manufacturers have begun to use microprocessors and other computer hardware as well as software in developing "intelligent" machines that can with the aid of a technician train patients, collect data, help with diagnosis, and conduct follow-ups.

Still another way of increasing the economy and cost-effectiveness of behavioral medicine techniques is to utilize home training procedures and self-instructions wherever possible. Surwit, Pilon, and Fenton (1978) and Keefe,

Surwit, and Pilon (1980) have demonstrated that home instruction in autogenic training can be as effective as biofeedback and other more cost-intensive procedures in the treatment of Raynaud's disease. These studies have led to the development of home training packages (e.g., Surwit, 1978, 1979), which allow the patient to do most of the training on his own at home, necessitating only brief follow-up visits to a professional office. While the relationship between professional change agent and the patient is still considered important, the operational definition of the process of therapeutic change inherent in Behavioral Medicine allows for division of labor that would have been unheard of in traditional psychosomatic approaches. Thus, behavioral approaches that prove to be effective can often be shown to be economically realistic alternatives to conventional medical treatment.

ASSESSMENT

It should go without saying that any patient who is being considered for behavioral treatment of a disease process should have first been thoroughly evaluated in a conventional medical fashion. Those patients whose diagnosis suggests that they will benefit from behavioral intervention are then candidates for further behavioral assessment. Once it is established that a patient is suffering from a disease process that may be amenable to behavioral treatment, the stage is set for behavioral assessment. Regardless of who carries out the behavioral assessment, the purpose of the assessment and treatment must be made clear to the patient at the very beginning. First of all, it should be understood by both the patient and the referral source that the decision to treat the patient's problem behaviorally does not imply that the patient is suffering from a psychiatric disorder. Too often it is assumed by all concerned that patients referred for such treatment have merely imaginary problems or are suffering from some neurosis. As noted in Chapter 1, this belief may have its origins in the traditional psychosomatic approach with its psychodynamic orientation to diagnosis and treatment. Patients being considered for behavioral treatment of disease need not be thought of as suffering from psychological difficulties. Rather, the selection of a behavioral treatment alternative is based upon efficacy, pathophysiology, cost-effectiveness, and other considerations, which should all be made clear to the patient before beginning.

Obtaining a Reliable Symptom Baseline

As Keefe, Kopel, and Gordon (1978) have pointed out, behavioral assessment is an integral part of behavioral intervention itself. One of the prime dif-

ferentiators between behavioral and other more traditional psychological approaches is the emphasis the behavioral approach places on empirical validity.
Thus, the natural first step in instituting a behavioral treatment is the collection of baseline data. It is important to get an accurate assessment of both the
physiological and the subjective aspects of the disease process in order to judge
whether a treatment is effective. Both objective and subjective information are
assessed because they tell us different things. While self-report of symptom
improvement is the ultimate goal toward which most therapeutic interventions
strive, patients' self-reports are notoriously inaccurate. Insomniacs, for example, typically exaggerate how long it takes them to fall asleep by as much as
400% (Freedman & Papsdorf, 1976; Rechtshoffen, 1968). Conversely, other
problems, such as migraine headaches, are often impossible to observe directly
because of their relative infrequent occurrence. Even when a patient's
headache occurs in the presence of a practitioner, the intensity of reported pain
is often difficult to correlate with objective indexes of muscle tension or blood
flow (Cox, Freundlich, & Myer, 1975). Miller and Dworkin (1977) noted that
a number of disorders that have been treated with biofeedback are chronic
conditions marked by fluctuations in symptom severity. Thus, patients are most
likely to seek treatment during periods of increased symptom activity. Spontaneous remissions of symptom severity may, therefore, coincide with the
course of treatment, and the improvement may be falsely attributed to the
success of behavioral intervention. In addition to the tendency of symptoms to
regress to a mean value, habituation of physiological responses to repeated
measurements presents an additional confounding circumstance. Surwit, Shapiro, and Good (1978) noted that, as a result of habituation to the stimulus
context of a behavioral treatment program for hypertension, patients' blood
pressures were shown to drop from 165/103 mm Hg to 139/88 mm Hg over two
baseline sessions. Once these baseline changes were factored out, further pressure decrements produced during training were shown to be only a few millimeters of mercury of magnitude. Similarly, Brady, Luborsky, and Kron (1974)
noted variations in systolic blood pressure ranging from 4 to 34 mm Hg during
evaluation and baseline periods. These fluctuations were much greater than
those attributable to metronome-conditioned relaxation treatment. Without
proper evaluation, exaggerated therapeutic efficacy would have been attributed
to these behavioral procedures in the treatment of hypertension. Problems of
subjective distortion on the part of the patient and symptom fluctuation resulting from the disease process itself can be minimized by instituting the reliable
method for collecting both baseline and in-treatment data. While the physiological and subjective aspects of some disorders, such as Raynaud's disease, seem
to correlate very nicely, the nature of other disorders may force the therapist to
focus on either physiology or subjective discomfort alone. For instance, in
monitoring headache frequency, subjective data of pain and discomfort is the

most important indicator of symptom severity. This can be monitored by having the patient rate his or her pain on a visual analog scale. In addition, requiring the patient to report prn medication intake, especially for analgesics, is also helpful in tracking symptom severity. For other disorders, such as hypertension, where few subjective symptoms exist, having the patients directly monitor their own physiology (blood pressure) on a regular basis is the most logical method of evaluation and assessment.

In addition to providing information that will help the clinician determine whether the treatment is having its desired effect, the process of behavioral assessment makes clear to the patient the logic behind the impending treatment program. Lynn and Freedman (1979) have also pointed out that it is useful to evaluate the patient's perception of the problem and the prospective treatment during the assessment phase.

> This is important because the patient may harbor doubts regarding participation in treatment and may entertain a variety of notions that may interfere with potential cooperation and involvement in therapy. For example, the person may indulge in fantasies of being shocked by the electrical equipment, entertain hopes for a magical or 'quick' cure and immediate symptom relief, or maintain a 'helpless, hopeless' attitude that precludes the ability to envision the positive therapeutic outcome [p. 453].

Developing a Functional Analysis

Whereas in many cases certain behavioral techniques such as relaxation can be effectively applied to the treatment of disease without clarification of the relationship of stress to symptom severity, it is always useful to assess the relationship between the symptom and the environmental stimuli that confronts the patient. The importance of this principle is illustrated in the case discussed by Schwartz (1973). A patient who was treated for essential hypertension during a week of treatment would lower his blood pressure by as much as 20 mm Hg. Over the weekend his pressure would become elevated again. The difficulty turned out to be that the patient liked to gamble at the racetrack on weekends and did so despite the fact that this activity was countertherapeutic. There is good evidence that certain schedules of reinforcement not only produce persistent behavior such as gambling but also can be seen as responsible for pressor reactions in otherwise normal animals (Benson, Herd, Morse, & Kelleher, 1970; Brady, 1958; Harris, Gilliam, Findley, & Brady, 1973). It is thus behaviorally naive to attempt to treat a disorder directly with biofeedback or relaxation where environmental contingencies are aggravating the problem. By performing a careful functional analysis, a program can be instituted to help deal with these environmental difficulties as part of the original treatment plan. On occasion behavioral assessment can be therapeutic in and of itself. Figure

9.1 shows graphs of blood pressures recorded by a patient during his waking hours. Therapy consisted of meeting with the patient on a weekly basis and discussing the environmental and situational precursors of pressor responses. Through a process of counseling, the patient was able to change his life-style in such a way as to reduce the number of stressful pressor situations and, by doing so, the mean systolic and diastolic blood pressure. Over a period of 3 months, the patient's pressure fluctuations diminished to the point where he could be considered essentially normotensive. Similar results have been observed by Engel (Note 1).

Meichenbaum (1976) points out that the initial assessment should include an explanation of cognitions that precede, accompany, and follow the symptom in addition to a situational analysis. Thus, a patient's symptoms can sometimes be seen to result from faulty cognitive assessments of otherwise benign situational events. In such a case, therapy could contain some sort of cognitive restructuring aimed at teaching the patient to reassess those situations to which his symptoms appear responsive. Once the relationship between situational stimuli, patients' cognitions, and a symptom is clarified to both the patient and therapist, then the patient can be taught to use different cognitive behaviors in response to the problematic stimulus situation. For instance, a Type A patient with hypertensive responses to such benign situations as a delay in a checkout line of a supermarket needs more than relaxation training to control blood pressure. A more effective technique might be to change the patients' reaction to the impending wait, instructing him to ask himself when he feels agitated by a line, "Am I really in a hurry? Maybe I should take this opportunity to browse through the magazines at the checkout counter?"

In addition to teaching the patient to use new and different cognitive strategies, it is sometimes useful to teach patients new overt behaviors in addition to various forms of relaxation. For instance, not all pressor responses are associated with Type A behavior. Sometimes patients who are inappropriately quiet and passive can be shown to respond with elevations in blood pressure to situations in which they fail to respond aggressively enough. In this case, assertiveness training may be more important than relaxation in producing decreases in blood pressure. In each case, the appropriate behavioral technique is dictated by the behavioral assessment itself.

Some investigators have used all these techniques together in a self-management coping skills approach. Mitchell and White (1977) have shown that patients suffering from chronic migraine headaches could benefit from a broad-spectrum behavioral treatment. Patients were given cassette tapes for self-instruction in relaxation, desensitization, and assertiveness training and taught to self-monitor stress and symptom frequency. Using a multiple baseline design, Mitchell and White were able to show that the interventions had an additive effect in reducing headache frequency. Their treatment model provides the patient with a series of behavioral techniques and teaches the patient to use these techniques as dictated by the patients' own behavioral analysis. Thus behavioral treatment of disease can be seen as a "technology of self-management" that emphasizes self-monitoring of a physiological response or symptom, learning when to implement self-control strategies most effectively, and self-reinforcement to maintain the practice of self-control (Blanchard & Epstein, 1978).

DEALING WITH MOTIVATIONAL DEFICITS

One of the weakest aspects of routine medical care is its lack of attention to motivational variables in dealing with patient compliance to prescribed treatment regimens. In any behavioral program, issues of motivation and compliance are obviously paramount to the success of the intervention. Shapiro and Surwit (1976, 1979) have commented extensively on the importance of patient motivation in any biofeedback treatment program.

A motivational problem encountered in the clinical application of behavioral techniques to the treatment of disease is that the symptom itself may be reinforcing to the patient. In other words, the disorder may have secondary gain. A striking example of this was reported by Surwit (1973). A patient who was involved in intensive biofeedback treatment for Raynaud's disease spontaneously expressed her ambivalence of "giving up" on her illness because she didn't know how to relate to other people without it. She was aware of using her Raynaud's disease as an excuse for a poor social life and dependent relationship with her mother. In this case, social training was carried out in an attempt to remedy the problem. Patients suffering from psychosomatic illnesses often use their well-known sensitivity to emotional situations to manipulate others (Lachman, 1972). A therapy based on voluntary control would tend to undermine their manipulations and consequently may not be seen as desirable by the patient. Although early models of behavior therapy tend to ignore the more subtle contingencies implicit in some behavioral problems, more recent writers are taking them into account (Kraft, 1972; Lazarus, 1971). In that some of these contingencies might not be known to the patient explicitly, they may be considered unconscious. A behavior therapy designed to treat a disorder supported by a secondary gain would therefore have to include techniques aimed at making up any social deficit left by the removal of the symptom. These might include setting up family contingencies or working on alternative means of social interaction. When the patient does not see the need for such additional procedures, insight-oriented psychotherapy may be called for as the first step.

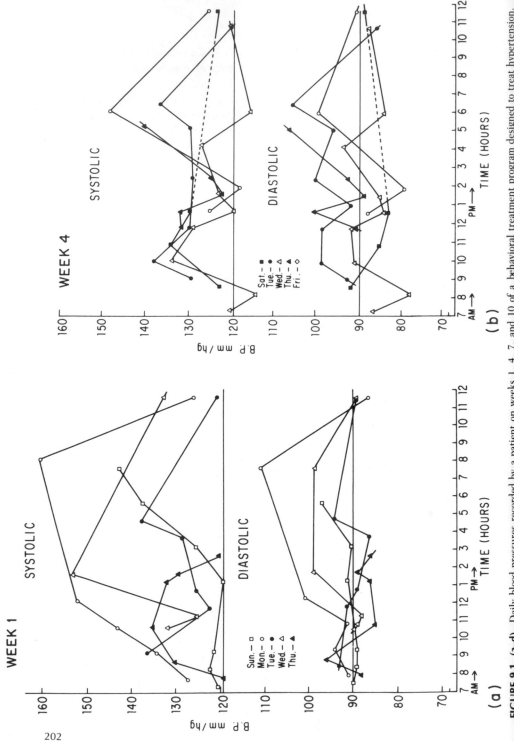

202

FIGURE 9.1. (a–d) Daily blood pressures recorded by a patient on weeks 1, 4, 7, and 10 of a behavioral treatment program designed to treat hypertension.

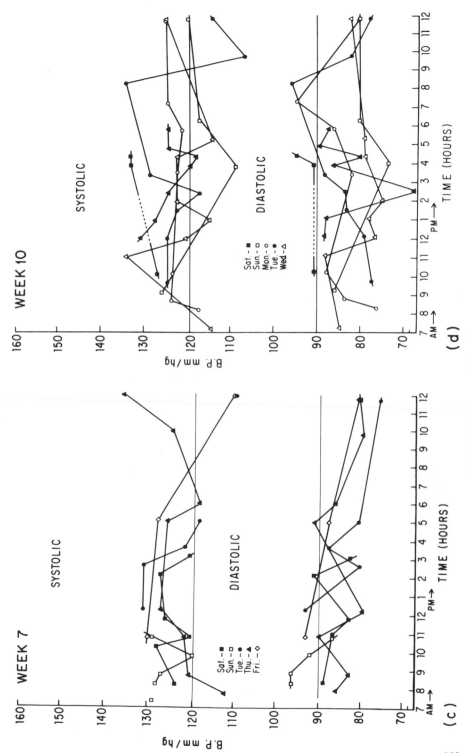

FIGURE 9.1. Continued from facing page.

TRANSFER OF TRAINING:
MAXIMIZING TREATMENT GAINS

An issue closely related to motivation, and equally important in the success-ful application of behavioral techniques to the treatment of disease, is transfer of training. Shapiro and Surwit (1976, 1979) have pointed out that learning techniques cannot be administered the way most medical treatments can. There is no reason to believe that, like radiation therapy or some surgical procedures, learned changes in physiology will produce sustained effects out-side of the training session without appropriate generalization procedures. It is completely logical that the patient may show perfect control of his or her problem during the training session and no control at home unless generaliza-tion procedures are employed. In basic research with normal subjects, inves-tigators have explored the use of intermittent reinforcement schedules as an aid to generalization (Green, 1966; Hefferline & Bruno, 1971; Shapiro & Crider, 1976; Shapiro & Watanabe, 1971; Weiss & Engel, 1971). Goldstein, Lopez, and Greenleaf (1979) isolated three general factors in the successful transfer of training from the clinical situation to the general environment. First, the greater the similarity between practice and test stimuli, the greater the amount of positive transfer to the actual situation. For example, the treatment of phobias is always most effective when the desensitization is done out in the real world. Lynn and Freedman (1979) point out that "while the traditional psychotherapeutic situation is far removed from the real world, the biofeedback environment is even more distant [p. 488]." In addition to the specificity of therapists and temporal factors in psychotherapy, biofeedback confronts the patient with an impressive array of machinery in an atmosphere that encour-ages relaxation and tuning out the "noise" of everyday life. Thus, the con-tingencies associated with controlling the physiological response in the labora-tory may be very different from those operating in the patient's real-life situation. Surwit, Pilon, and Fenton (1978) and Keefe et al. (1980) have shown that training patients to practice voluntary vasodilatation at home using brief minipractices throughout the day appears to be the most essential element in the effective behavioral treatment of Raynaud's disease.

The second important element in transfer of training from the clinical situation to the patient's real world has to do with frequency of practice. The likelihood that a response will be available is very clearly a function of its prior usage. The more often we repeat a behavior—that is, the more we practice it—the better we are at producing it. One of the basic principles of learning theory is that overlearned responses tend to be well remembered. Overlearning is the procedure whereby learning is extended beyond the point necessary to produce initial changes in behavior. This implies more than the old adage of practice makes perfect (implying that one should practice until one gets it right). Mandler (1954) and Mandler and Hinneman (1956) have shown that it is important to be able to perform a response without error. Thus, it is practice of a perfect response that tends to reinforce its transfer to other situations. Patient manuals have been devised for progressive relaxation and autogenic training that specifically emphasize frequent practice (e.g., Surwit, 1978, 1979). Patients are advised to practice relaxation or vasodilatation briefly for between 30 sec and 1 min up to 20 times a day. To aid them in this process, they are given instructions in various methods to key themselves to remember to practice. One such method involves placing little colored dots in salient places, such as on the telephone, the refrigerator, the bathroom mirror, the front door, which would serve as a reminder to practice the newly developed habit. The use of progressive muscle relaxation and autogenic training tapes that are fairly portable and allow the patient to practice at home is another way of maximizing response availability.

Finally, transfer of training can be facilitated by maximizing stimulus variability. While the sheer number of correct responses will aid in allowing the patient to generalize a newly learned response to other situations, the situations in which the response is practiced also help determine the durability of the new behavior. Group therapy is perhaps the most common systematic attempt to provide stimulus variability in therapy. However, in the treatment of disease states, many of the procedures utilized for maximizing response variability will also maximize stimulus variability. If patients are instructed to practice the new response in as many different situations as many times a day as they can, then both such goals will be reinforced. Clinicians should remember that new healthy physiological responses will not automatically generalize from the clinical situation to the real world unless this generalization is intentionally and systematically programmed. The techniques listed here to help patients remember to practice a new skill will also lead them to practice under variable stimulus conditions. In summary, effective behavior change depends upon practicing correctly, frequently, and in varied stimulus conditions similar to those encountered in everyday life.

BEHAVIORAL COMPLIANCE WITH MEDICAL REGIMENS

Another area in which behavior plays a central role in medicine involves patient compliance with conventional modes of medical treatment. Although patient compliance is the key component in behavior modification programs designed to treat disease, it is also an essential factor in the efficacy of almost all outpatient therapeutic regimens. It is often forgotten that behavioral change is an integral part in the administration of all successful medical interventions. Pill taking is a behavior just as practicing relaxation is. Although patients do not have to learn how to take medication, there is no reason to assume that medication-taking behavior will persist in a regular fashion unless it is programmed to do so. Adherence to more complex medical regimens that involve discomfort, time-consuming operations, or complex behavior change (e.g., diet change) are less likely to be followed unless the factors that reinforce and maintain new behaviors are taken into account.

Blackwell (1979) has summarized the present state of knowledge concerning the relationship of the nature of medical treatment and patient compliance. These factors are listed in Table 9.1. With respect to compliance with drug regimens, one can see that the factors mitigating against compliance include complexity of the regimen. Although Blackwell notes that the recent emphasis on once daily regimens is not supported by much hard data, he cites Ayd (1972), who in reviewing a series of unpublished reports noted that, whereas 30% of the patients on a twice daily regimen failed to take their medication, 70% failed to take medication when their regimen called for a three or four times daily

TABLE 9.1
Factors That Affect Adherence

Factors that increase adherence		Factors that decrease adherence	
Factor	Number of studies in favor	Factor	Number of studies in favor
Patient views disease as serious	7	Complexity of regimen	12
Family stability	7	Behavior change required of patient	4
Compliance with other aspects	5	Clinic waiting time	4
Patient satisfaction	1	Block versus individual booking	2
Close supervision by physician	4	Painful therapy	2
Private practice versus clinic	2	Psychological problems	2
Patient expectations met	2	Low frustration tolerance	2
Physician accepts patient	2	Nervous symptoms	2
Mother agrees with physician	2	Working mothers	2
Degree of disability	2		

Source: From B. Blackwell. Treatment adherence in hypertension. *American Journal of Pharmacology*, 1976, *148*, 75–85, 614.

administration. The number of the drugs taken also affects compliance with drug regimens. Blackwell (1979) notes in his review of the literature that, while the data are scanty on the affects of multiple dosage on compliance, there is reason to believe that compliance suffers in such a treatment regimen. He points out, however, that it is not clear whether or not a failure of patients to comply with multiple-drug regimens can be attributed to poor compliance or simply to poor understanding.

A variable that appears to mitigate for compliance to a therapeutic regimen is how seriously a patient views his or her illness. Hulka, Kupper, Cassel, Efird, and Burdette (1975) have shown that patients taking gastrointestinal drugs and tranquilizers make more scheduling errors than those patients taking medication for serious cardiac or diabetic conditions. From a behavioral standpoint, it is obvious that the contingencies for accurate compliance are much clearer for the latter group of patients than for the former.

Dunbar, Marshall, and Hovell (1979) reviewed strategies that have been designed to improve patient compliance with medical regimens. They have identified six behavioral strategies that have been employed in increasing patient compliance.

The simplest and most straightforward procedure in attempting to maintain patient compliance is to use *periodic reminders*. Brigg and Mudd (1968) and Turner and Vernon (1976) have both reported that reminders help prevent appointment breaking in patients who are undergoing psychological counseling. Reminders have also been used to improve medication compliance. Lima, Nazarin, Charney, and Lahti (1976) conducted a three-group controlled outcome comparison study with outpatients undergoing antimicrobial therapy. One patient group received prescription labels with a clock face upon which the hours of administration were circled. The second group received special labels containing directions for administration that could be placed away from the medication in an obvious place. The third group served as a control, and the medication was conventionally labeled with no attempt to provide an additional reminder. Both groups that received reminders did better than the controls, although the compliance of these two groups did not differ from each other.

A second technique thought to improve compliance is *tailoring*. It has been found in behavioral studies that behavior modification procedures work most effectively when they are tailored to the needs of the patient. Best (1975) has shown that the efficacy of attitude change procedures in a smoking withdrawal program depends upon how they are utilized with each individual patient. Whereas attitude change procedures tend to be more effective with less motivated patients after abstinence is achieved, highly motivated patients profit more from these procedures when they are introduced early on. Hallburg (1970) demonstrated that tailoring the medication regimens of elderly patients to their routines and particular needs reduced by half the number of errors that patients made in taking their medication. Haynes, Sackett, Gibson, Taylor, Hackett, Roberts, and Johnson (1976) demonstrated that by matching medication administration to the times and places of the patients daily habits, a significant improvement in compliance in otherwise noncompliant populations undergoing antihypertensive therapy could be achieved. However, the treatment group also received increased supervision and home blood pressure measurement in addition to the tailoring procedure.

Still another technique widely used in behavior therapy for increasing compliance to behavioral change regimens is *contracting*. Contracting refers to a procedure in which the therapist makes a contract with the patient specifying particular contingencies that will occur based on the patient's behavior. The contract can specify particular rewards that the patient will allow himself to indulge in following the completion of the desired behavior (e.g., after he takes his pill, he will turn on the television) or can involve a relationship between the behavior or the practitioner and the compliance of the patient (e.g., after he has taken his pills, he will be able to come in for another appointment). Mahoney and Thoresen (1974) have listed five guidelines for developing a successful behavioral contract:

1. The contract should be fair to both the patient and the therapist.
2. The terms of the contract should be very clear.
3. The contract should be generally positive.
4. The procedure should be systematic and consistent.
5. At least one other person should be involved in the contract.

The utility of contracting to improve compliance with medication administration, weight loss, and stress management in patients undergoing blood pressure control has been demonstrated by Steckel and Swain (1977). In this study the contract involved the delivery of inexpensive tangible reinforcements to patients who had met specific goals spelled out in the contract. Bigelow, Strickler, Leisbon, and Griffiths (1976) worked with patients undergoing disulfiram therapy for alcoholism. They were required to place a financial security deposit with the investigators. Ingestion of disulfiram was done at the clinic, and patients had to report to the clinic for 14 days and then on alternate days for a minimum of 3 months. Failure to report to the clinic and take the medication resulted in forfeit of the deposit. Using breatholyzer readings as a dependent variable, subject abstinence from alcohol was found to last at least four times longer using the contracts than it had previously lasted before the contracts had been instituted. Interestingly, 70% of the subjects who participated in the study volunteered for a second contract after the initial period was over.

Shaping is the building of a new behavior by reinforcing successive approximations of the desired behavior. It is assumed that it is often unrealistic to require patients to produce a behavior that is not currently in their repertoire.

Thus, assigning a patient who has never taken medication to a four times daily regimen is less likely to succeed initially than asking the patient to begin taking one pill a day and gradually increasing the regimen up to a full dose. The use of shaping also has the advantage of decreasing side effects of medication (Brosens, Robertson, & Von Assche, 1974; Seybold & Drachman, 1974).

Self-monitoring has also been shown to be useful in various kinds of behavior change. Self-monitoring refers to observing and recording ones own behavior. Keefe, Kopel, and Gordon (1978) noted that self-monitoring procedures can in themselves produce substantial behavior change. The most common form of self-monitoring involves the daily use of a scale to control weight. Indeed such programs as Weight Watchers have long avocated multiple self-monitoring procedures for controlling weight. Patients are instructed in calorie counting as well as in estimating energy expenditure and recording these variables as a means of helping to regulate weight. Dunbar *et al.* (1979) cite a doctoral thesis by Dunbar in which self-monitoring of medication was used in a controlled study of poor compliers. Although compliance was not significantly altered by a self-monitoring procedure during the experimental treatment, patients in the experimental condition made continuous and progressive gains that were obvious at a 6-month follow-up.

The sixth technique for increasing patient compliance is *reinforcement*. In Chapter 1 we reviewed the basic paradigms of learning. As noted, a primary postulate of behavior is that any behavior that is followed by consequences perceived as rewarding will have an increasing likelihood of being repeated. When the reward of something consists of something new and positive, it is called positive reinforcement. If the reward consists of the cessation of an ongoing negative or aversive event, we then refer to the process as negative reinforcement. Praising a patient for good compliance is an example of positive reinforcement. When a patient complies with a regimen because it relieves pain, he is being negatively reinforced for doing so. Reinforcement of either type is most effective if it follows the desired behavior closely in time.

This simple principle has profound implications for compliance with health care regimens. Activities that are punished or ignored tend to diminish in frequency, whereas those that have clear, immediate, and favorable consequences become stronger. Shapiro and Surwit (1976, 1979) have repeatedly pointed out that the ability of a treatment to reduce uncomfortable symptomatology is an important determinant in patient compliance with behavioral regimens in the treatment of disease. Dunbar *et al.* (1979) have noted that this is equally important in the implementation of more conventional medical regimens.

Where positive or negative reinforcement is not naturally built into a treatment regimen by its ability to make the patient feel better, then sometimes reinforcement needs to be programmed artificially. Bellak, Rozensky, and

Schwartz (1974) and Mahoney, Moura, and Wade (1973) have demonstrated that programmed positive reinforcement can improve compliance to a weight reduction regimen, which is in itself aversive. Mahoney et al. have also noted that positive reinforcement is superior to applying aversive consequences as a means of increasing compliance. As Dunbar et al. (1979) note, the administration of reinforcement can be implemented by people other than the clinical staff. Reinforcement for compliance implemented by fellow workers, family, and friends can be an effective component in an antihypertension program (Alderman & Schoenbaum, 1975). Behavioral programs can also be effectively carried out by parents and teachers (Ryback & Surwit, 1971). Regardless of who the primary change agent is, the efficacy of positive reinforcement depends on the proper relationship between behavior and consequences. This relationship is the single most important principle of behavioral control and is crucial to the successful outcome of any behavioral intervention.

REFERENCE NOTE

1. Engel, B. T. Personal communication, March 1981.

REFERENCES

Alderman, M., & Schoenbaum, E. Detection and treatment of hypertension at the work site. *New England Journal of Medicine*, 1975, 293, 65–68.

Ayd, F. J., Jr. (Ed.). Once-a-day neuroleptic and tricyclic antidepressant therapy. *International Drug Therapy Newsletter*, 1972, 7, 33–40.

Bellak, A. S., Rozensky, R., & Schwartz, J. A. A comparison of two forms of self-monitoring in a behavioral weight reduction program. *Behavior Therapy*, 1974, 5, 523–530.

Benson, H., Herd, J. A., Morse, W. H., & Kelleher, R. T. Behaviorally induced hypertension in the squirrel monkey. *Clinical Research*, 1970, 26–27 (Supp. 1), 21–26.

Best, J. A. Tailoring smoking withdrawal procedures to personality and motivational differences. *Journal of Consulting and Clinical Psychology*, 1975, 43, 1–8.

Bigelow, G., Strickler, D., Leisbon, I., & Griffiths, R. Maintaining disulfiram ingestion among outpatient alcoholics: A security-deposit contingency contacting procedure. *Behavior Research and Therapy*, 1976, 14, 378–381.

Blackwell, B. Treatment adherence in hypertension. *American Journal of Pharmacology*, 1976, 148, 75–85.

Blackwell, B. The drug regimen and treatment compliance. In R. B. Haynes, D. W. Taylor, & D. L. Sackett (Eds.), *Compliance in health care*. Baltimore: Johns Hopkins Press, 1979.

Blanchard, E. B., & Epstein, L. H. *A biofeedback primer,* Reading, Mass.: Addison-Wesley, 1978.

Brady, J. B., Luborsky, L., & Kron, R. E. Blood pressure reduction in patients with essential hypertension through metronome-conditional relaxation: A preliminary report. *Behavior Therapy*, 1974, *5*, 203–209.

Brady, J. B. Ulcers in "executive" monkeys. *Scientific American*, 1958, *199*, 95–103.

Brigg, E. H., & Mudd, E. H. An exploration of methods to reduce broken first appointments. *Family Coordinator*, 1968, *17*, 41–46.

Brosens, I. A., Robertson, W. B., & Von Assche, F. A. Assessment of incremental dosage regimen of combined oestrogen-progestogen oral contraceptive. *British Medical Journal*, 1974, *4*, 643–645.

Cox, D. J., Freundlich, A., & Myer, R. G. Differential effectiveness of electromyographic feedback, verbal relaxation instructions, and medication placebo with tension headaches. *Journal of Consulting and Clinical Psychology*, 1975, *43*, 897–899.

Dunbar, J. M., Marshall, G. D., & Hovell, M. F. Behavioral strategies for improving compliance. In R. B. Haynes, O. W. Taylor, & D. L. Sackett (Eds.), *Compliance in health care*. Baltimore: Johns Hopkins Press, 1979.

Freedman, R., & Papsdorf, J. D. Biofeedback and progress in relaxation of sleep-onset insomnia: A controlled, all night investigation. *Biofeedback and Self Regulation*, 1976, *3*, 253–272.

Goldstein, A. P., Lopez, M., & Greenleaf, D. O. Introduction to A. P. Goldstein & F. H. Kanfer (Eds.), *Maximizing treatment gains: Transfer enhancement in psychotherapy*. New York: Academic Press, 1979.

Green, W. A. Operant conditioning of the GSR using partial reinforcement. *Psychological Reports*, 1966, *19*, 571–578.

Hallburg, J. C. Teaching patients self-care. *Nursing Clinics of North America*, 1970, *5*, 223–231.

Harris, A. H., Gilliam, W. J., Findley, J. D., & Brady, J. B. Instrumental conditioning of large magnitudinal, daily, 12-hour blood pressure elevations in the baboon. *Science*, 1973, *182*, 175–177.

Haynes, R. B., Sackett, D. L., Gibson, E. S., Taylor, O. W., Hackett, B. C., Roberts, R. S., & Johnson, A. L. Improvement of medication compliance in uncontrolled hypertension. *Lancet*, 1976, *1*, 1265–1268.

Hefferline, R. F., & Bruno, L. J. J. The psychophysiology of private events. In A. Jacobs & L. Sachs (Eds.), *The psychology of private events*. New York: Academic Press, 1971.

Hulka, B., Kupper, L., Cassel, J., Efird, R., & Burdette, J. Medication use and misuse: Physician–patient discrepancies. *Journal of Chronic Disease*, 1975, *28*, 7–21.

Keefe, F. J., Kopel, S., & Gordon, S. *A practical guide to behavioral assessment*. New York: Springer Publ., 1978.

Keefe, F. J., Surwit, R. S., & Pilon, R. M. Biofeedback, autogenic training and progressive relaxation in the treatment of Raynaud's disease: A comparative study. *Journal of Applied Behavior Analysis*, 1980, *13*, 3–11.

Kraft, T. The use of behavior therapy in a psychotherapeutic contest. In A. A. Lazarus (Ed.), *Clinical behavior therapy*. New York: Brunner/Mazel, 1972.

Lachman, S. J. *Psychosomatic disorders: A behavioral interpretation*. New York: Wiley, 1972.

Lanyon, R. I., & Lanyon, B. P. *Behavior therapy: A clinical introduction*. Reading, Mass.: Addison-Wesley, 1978.

Lazarus, A. *Behavior therapy and beyond*. New York: McGraw-Hill, 1971.

Lima, J., Nazarian, L., Charney, E., & Lahti, C. Compliance with short term antimicrobial therapy: Some techniques that help. *Pediatrics*, 1976, *57*, 383–386.

Lynn, S. J., & Freedman, R. Transfer and evaluation of biofeedback. In A. P. Goldstein & F. H. Kanfer (Eds.), *Maximizing treatment and gains: Transfer enhancement in psychotherapy*. New York: Academic Press, 1979.

Mahoney, M. J., Moura, N. G. M., & Wade, T. C. The relative efficacy of self-rewards, self-punishment and self-monitoring techniques for weight loss. *Journal of Consulting and Clinical Psychology*, 1973, *40*, 404–407.

Mahoney, M. J., & Thoresen, C. E. *Self-control: Power to the person.* Monterey, Cal.: Brooks-Cole, 1974.

Mandler, G. Transfer of training as a function of degree of response over learning. *Journal of Experimental Psychology,* 1954, *47,* 411–417.

Mandler, G., & Hinneman, S. H. Effect of over learning of a verbal response on transfer of training. *Journal of Experimental Psychology,* 1956, *52,* 39–46.

Meichenbaum, D. Cognitive factors in biofeedback therapy. *Biofeedback and Self-Regulation,* 1976, *1,* 216.

Miller, N. E., & Dworkin, B. R. Critical issues in the therapeutic application of biofeedback. In G. E. Schwartz & J. Beatty (Eds.), *Biofeedback: Theory and research.* New York: Academic Press, 1977.

Mitchell, K. R., & White, R. G. Behavioral self-management: An application to the problem of migraine headaches. *Behavior Therapy,* 1977, *8,* 213–221.

Rechtshoffen, A. Polygraphic aspects of insomnia. In H. Gesteaut, E. Lugaresi, G. Berti-Ceroni, & C. Coccagna (Eds.), *The abnormalities of sleep in man.* Bologna: Aulo Goggi Editore, 1968.

Ryback, D., & Surwit, R. S. Sub-professional behavior modification in the development of token-reinforcement systems in increasing academic motivation and achievement. *Child Study Journal,* 1971, *1,* 52–68.

Schwartz, G. E. Biofeedback as therapy: Some theoretical and practical issues. *American Psychologist,* 1973, *28,* 666–673.

Seybold, M. E., & Drachman, D. B. Gradually increasing doses of prednisone in myasthenia gravis. *New England Journal of Medicine,* 1974, *290,* 81–84.

Shapiro, D., & Crider, A. Operant electrodermal conditioning under multiple schedule of reinforcement. *Psychophysiology,* 1967, *4,* 168–175.

Shapiro, D., & Surwit, R. S. Learned control of physiological function and disease. In H. Leitenberg (Ed.), *Handbook of behavior modification and behavior therapy.* Englewood Cliffs, N.J.: Prentice-Hall, 1976.

Shapiro, D., & Surwit, R. S. Biofeedback. In O. Pomerlean & J. P. Brady (Eds.), *Behavioral medicine: Theory and practice.* Baltimore: Williams & Wilkins, 1979.

Shapiro, D., & Watanabe, T. Timing characteristics of operant electrodermal modification: Fixed interval effects. *Japanese Psychological Research,* 1971, *13,* 123–130.

Steckel, S. B., & Swain, M. A. Contracting with patients to improve compliance. *Journal of the American Hospital Association,* 1977, *51,* 81–84.

Surwit, R. S. Biofeedback: A possible treatment for Raynaud's disease. In L. Birk (Ed.), *Biofeedback: Behavioral medicine.* New York: Grune & Stratton, 1973.

Surwit, R. S. *Autogenic training manual.* Durham, N.C.: Duke Univ., 1978.

Surwit, R. S. *Progressive relaxation training manual.* Durham, N.C.: Duke Univ., 1979.

Surwit, R. S., & Keefe, F. J. Frontalis EMG biofeedback: An electronic panacea? *Behavior Therapy,* 1978, *9,* 779–792.

Surwit, R. S., Pilon, R. N., & Fenton, C. H. Behavioral treatment of Raynaud's disease. *Journal of Behavioral Medicine,* 1978, *1,* 323–335.

Surwit, R. S., Shapiro, D., & Good, M. I. Comparison of cardiovascular biofeedback, neuromuscular biofeedback, and meditation in the treatment of borderline essential hypertension. *Journal of Consulting and Clinical Psychology,* 1978, *46,* 252–263.

Turner, A. J., & Vernon, J. C. Prompts to increase attendance in a community mental-health center. *Journal of Applied Behavior Analysis,* 1976, *9,* 141–145.

Weiss, T., & Engel, B. T. Operant conditioning of heart rate in patients with premature ventricular contractions. *Psychosomatic Medicine,* 1971, *33,* 301–321.

Author Index

Numbers in italics refer to the pages on which the complete references are listed.

Subject Index